Making Your Data Work

TOOLS AND TEMPLATES

FOR EFFECTIVE ANALYSIS

Kenneth R. Rohde

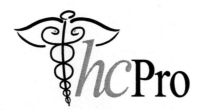

Making Your Data Work: Tools and Templates for Effective Analysis is published by HCPro, Inc.

Copyright © 2008 HCPro, Inc.

All rights reserved. Printed in the United States of America.   5   4   3   2   1

ISBN 978-1-60146-145-2

HCPro, Inc., provides information resources for the healthcare industry.

HCPro, Inc., is not affiliated in any way with The Joint Commission, which owns the JCAHO and Joint Commission trademarks.

Kenneth R. Rohde, Author

Mary Stevens, Senior Managing Editor

Brian Driscoll, Executive Editor

John Novack, Group Publisher

Patrick Campagnone, Cover Designer

Mike Mirabello, Senior Graphic Artist

Michael Roberto, Layout Artist

Audrey Doyle, Copyeditor

Lauren Rubenzahl, Proofreader

Darren Kelly, Books Production Supervisor

Susan Darbyshire, Art Director

Claire Cloutier, Production Manager

Jean St. Pierre, Director of Operations

Advice given is general. Readers should consult professional counsel for specific legal, ethical, or clinical questions.

Arrangements can be made for quantity discounts. For more information, contact:

HCPro, Inc.
P.O. Box 1168
Marblehead, MA 01945
Telephone: 800/650-6787 or 781/639-1872
Fax: 781/639-2982
E-mail: *customerservice@hcpro.com*

Visit HCPro at its World Wide Web sites:
www.hcpro.com and *www.hcmarketplace.com*

12/2007
21340

Contents

Contents

Figure List

About the author

Kenneth R. Rohde

Kenneth R. Rohde is a senior consultant for The Greeley Company, a division of HCPro, Inc. He brings more than 27 years of experience in quality and organizational management to his work with hospitals, medical centers, and industrial facilities across the country.

Rohde's roles in performance improvement and project management make him uniquely qualified to assist medical staffs and hospital leaders in developing solutions to their toughest challenges. He instructs, speaks, and consults in the areas of error reduction strategies, root cause analysis, improving performance through process simplification, error reduction through effective procedure writing, apparent cause analysis, engineering effectiveness and error reduction, failure modes and effects analysis, effective data collection, analysis and trending, patient safety evaluation and improvement, change management, corrective action program evaluation and redesign, human performance evaluations, and procedure error reduction. Rohde also specializes in technology-based approaches to preventing human errors and analyzing performance data.

Prior to joining The Greeley Company, Rohde served as director for Performance Improvement International and director of corrective actions process at Westinghouse Electric Company. He has also participated in or managed projects to improve business effectiveness and business development for healthcare, nuclear power, and manufacturing facilities around the globe.

Rohde is also the author of *Failure Modes and Effect Analysis: Templates and Tools to Improve Patient Safety*, published by HCPro.

Rohde holds a B.S. in mechanical engineering from University of Hawaii.

Introduction

Data surrounds us, and every day it influences what we do in our lives. The trick is to make sure that the data serves us and that we don't become slaves to our data.

Think about traveling cross country in your car. You glance at the dashboard and sample a variety of data related to speed, gas, and engine temperature on a regular basis. If you are a relatively cautious driver, you use that data to change your behavior. If the gas tank is getting low, you fill it up. If the speed is creeping up, you slow down. There is a direct relationship between the data you collect as you drive and *how* you drive. This is the feedback or control loop that makes you a good driver.

But you can become overwhelmed with the data as well. The navigation system is talking to you and urging that you turn left, while your "copilot," who is reading the map, is telling you to go straight ahead. The low-fuel light is blinking, and voices from the back seat are providing input regarding the need for food and bathrooms. With too much data, your stress level goes up, and you can't decide what to pay attention to and what to ignore. Soon you want to just shut it all out and make a decision—any decision. The data that started out as such a useful and vital part of your safe driving is now turning on you and becoming a distraction—or, perhaps even worse, is making you drive in an unsafe manner.

Data in the healthcare environment can be a lot like the data on a cross-country car trip. We know that the data contains useful information that can help us get better and keep our patients and employees safe. We also know that the data will help us to be more productive and evidence-based and that it will help the organization succeed.

But soon we find that we are spending more of our time and money collecting more and more data, some of it useful and some of it just required. The data "noise level" starts to go up, and we can't do the analysis we would like to do to help people change their behaviors based on the data, so we just send it out and hope for the best. Sometimes, in the worst case, we find we are spending so much of our time and resources collecting, caring for, and feeding our data that we do not have enough time to take care of our patients—and that once-wonderful data has now become a distraction and maybe even a patient safety hazard.

So, what to do? The goal of this book is to help you start to get your data back under control and to help you get it back in its rightful place: serving you and facilitating your decision-making.

This book will focus on the areas that I have found through my consulting work to be the quickest and most productive ways to help a facility or team get its data back under control, separate valuable information from background noise, and begin to take data analysis to a higher level.

The following chapters will provide concise explanations of why data is so important to healthcare today, how to gather the most useful data for any project, and how best to present it to audiences at all levels, from the Board of Directors to unit managers. The accompanying figures show you your options, and the tips throughout the book can help you "get to the point" of these concepts.

In addition, the glossary at the end of this book and the resources included on the companion CD-ROM will help your teams get a handle on good data-gathering, presentations, and analysis.

So take a deep breath, and let's get started.

CHAPTER

1

Why Data Is So Important

What is data?

Data can be defined as factual information that forms the basis for our reasoning, discussions, and decisions. But that definition assumes that some preprocessing has occurred because data can also be thought of as collected information from our senses or measuring devices that may be either irrelevant or useful, depending on how we process it.

In the paper-and-pencil era, data had a way of being self-controlled—we just couldn't manage too much data, so we were more cautious about what we collected, stored, and analyzed.

In today's digital era, we have tremendously powerful tools for managing data, but we can also collect every trivial piece of information, store it, graph it in six different colors, and e-mail it to hundreds of coworkers.

What, then, is a realistic goal for the collection and use of our data? Why do we do it?

Goal: Use data to cause positive change

Effective data needs to be able to cause change. It needs to be an integral part of the "control loop" for your facility. If the data does not validate or change behaviors, it is not very useful and probably is resulting in the expenditure of time and effort with limited value.

Data that does not validate or change our behavior is not very useful.

Data also needs to serve us, not make our goals harder to achieve. So who needs to be able to use data effectively? In one way or another, we *all* need to be able to effectively use data. Often the Quality and Performance Improvement, Infection Control, and Risk Management departments are key collectors and managers of data, but the real value of data extends from the clinical and non-clinical frontline all the way through the board.

Who needs to understand data?

The secret to making your data useful throughout the organization is to recognize that not everyone wants or needs the same data (see Figure 1.1). Although we might be tempted to provide the board of directors with a 150-page data report each quarter, that may not be useful if board members get to spend only 15 minutes looking at the report before they meet and then hear a 20-minute overview presentation. That's lots of data—but probably not likely to validate actions or cause change.

Likewise, a comprehensive presentation to the dietary group on the current status of core measures might be interesting, but it probably will not validate their actions or cause change within their department.

One of the key concepts we will discuss in Chapter 4 is the ability to roll up and zoom in on data. This keeps the data linked together and ensures that the detailed inputs from particular departments are part of the big picture, but it also allows the data to be rolled up into more useful summaries as we present our findings to people and departments higher up in the organization.

FIGURE **1.1**   Match the data to the needs of the user

User	Data Need
Board of directors	• Is the organization meeting our highest-level goals and commitments to the community, employees, and stakeholders? (Stakeholder data) • Does the data validate that we are on an acceptable path, or does it indicate that the organization needs to change direction?
Senior leadership	• Are we meeting our long-term strategic and financial goals? (Strategic data) • Are there major areas of emerging concern that need to be addressed before they turn into major problems? (Early warning)
Directors	• Are we meeting our shorter-term tactical goals this month? This year?
Managers and supervisors	• Are we meeting our daily and weekly operational goals? • What can we do within our department to be safer and more efficient or to provide higher levels of patient and employee satisfaction?
All employees	• How is my job going? • What are the risks I need to look out for? • Is the organization healthy?

The data cycle

The data cycle starts with data collection and storage of that data in such a way that it can be retrieved. Then we need to analyze, mine, and listen to the data so that we can understand what it is telling us. Finally, we need to present and share the data. Figure 1.2 depicts this data cycle.

FIGURE **1.2**   The data cycle must result in an appropriate response

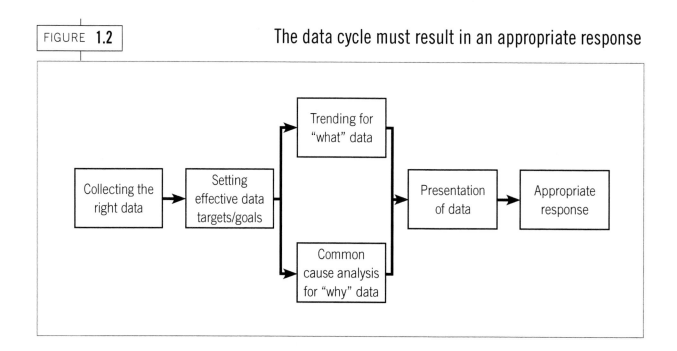

If the data cycle is working well, there is a strong connection between the data that is collected and the system's response. This is called a ***closed control loop*** because the data feeds from the behavior and then validates it or causes the behavior to change; then that behavior feeds back into the data, which then adjusts the behavior, and so on.

A *"broken" control loop* happens when we collect data and it has no impact on behavior, or we are measuring the wrong thing so that a change in behavior is not reflected back into the data. Either way, the loop doesn't work. Not only have we wasted all our data collection efforts, but we probably have a process that may be "out of control" or even unsafe.

Figure 1.3 compares these two types of control loops.

FIGURE 1.3   Closed control loops versus broken control loops

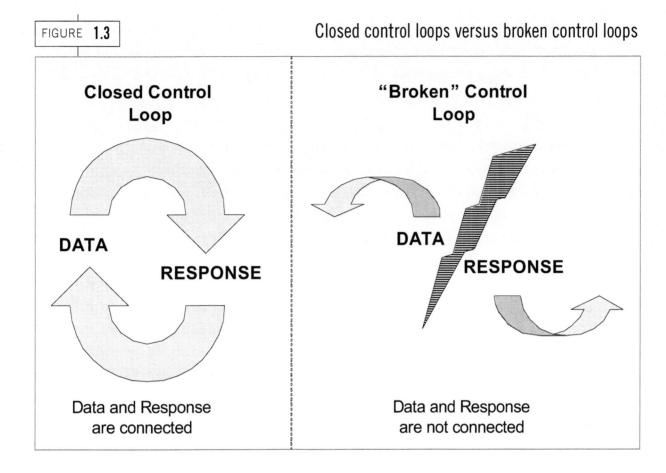

Closed Control Loop

DATA

RESPONSE

Data and Response
are connected

"Broken" Control Loop

DATA   RESPONSE

Data and Response
are not connected

Thinking about control loops

Using your electric blanket: A control loop example

A classic example of a control loop is the process of maintaining the temperature of an electric blanket on a bed. A thermostat in the blanket measures the temperature (*data*) and then compares it to the desired temperature (*setpoint*) that the user selects via a controller on the bedside table. Then, depending on the relationship of the blanket temperature (*data*) to the desired temperature (*setpoint*), the controller turns the blanket on or off (*response*).

This can be considered a closed control loop if the electric blanket warms up, the thermostat measures the new temperature (*data*), and the loop continues to work—the user stays at a comfortable temperature all night long.

A closed control loop is the ideal situation, but sometimes a closed control loop is hard to achieve. Take, for example, an electric blanket that has two controllers: one for each side of the bed. What happens if you mix up the controllers and the controller for the right-hand side of the bed ends up controlling the left-hand side, and vice versa?

In such a scenario, the person on the right-hand side gets cold, so he or she turns up what is thought to be the correct controller. That doesn't do anything to that person's side of the blanket, but it does turn up the other side. Now that other person starts to get hot and reaches over and turns down his or her controller. That has no effect on the temperature on the left side of the bed, but it makes the other side of the bed even colder. This keeps going until one person is sweltering and the other person is freezing.

In that example, both of the control loops are "broken," and the responses taken are not connected to the data. In the end, we have a mess.

Can broken control loops happen to your hospital or care facility? Absolutely! For example, one senior vice president might look at a data report and adjust his or her "control" (e.g., finance), which then affects another area that he or she did not recognize (e.g., staffing, patient safety, and purchasing). Then another senior vice president looks at different data and makes another adjustment that he or she thinks will improve the situation, but in reality it causes another department's data to change. Before you know it, both senior vice presidents feel like things are out of control.

Control loops are called that for a reason—they determine how we manage and control our organizations and processes, and they depend on having good data. That means we need to do an excellent job collecting, analyzing, and presenting our data so that the data not only causes change but also changes things appropriately.

Just like pieces of equipment, our key processes are often control loops. For example, we can look at the entire performance improvement/quality process as a big control loop (see Figure 1.4). We set expectations or goals and then collect data to compare against those expectations. Then, based on the differences between our expectations and the data we collect, we identify gaps and design improvements if necessary. Next, the improvements are implemented, and we expect to see a change

FIGURE 1.4   Performance improvement is a control loop

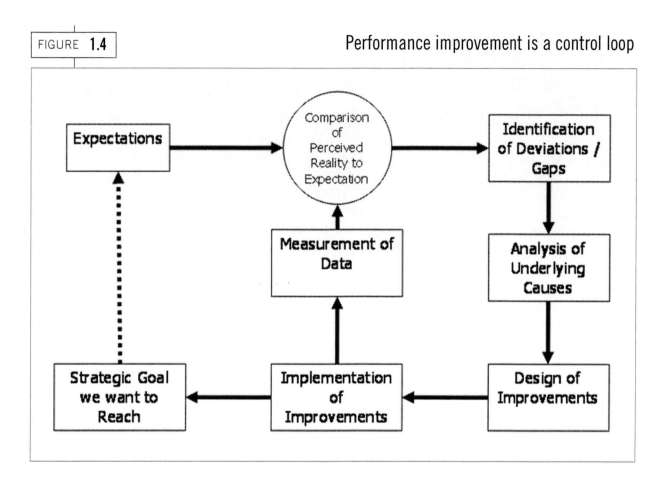

in the data. If we do see a change and the change is in the right direction, we are comfortable that we have made a real performance improvement.

If the data we collect is not connected to the expectations or the response, or if the data is poorly collected or analyzed, we can have a significant breakdown in the performance improvement process. Failures in our performance improvement control loop can result in known problems not being fixed, increases in patient and employee safety events, regulatory or accreditation problems, and ultimately, challenges to the survival of the organization.

Our ability to recognize the ways a control loop fails is a vital part of managing the organization and keeping our processes under control.

Typical failures in a control loop

Good data managers and analysts need to understand how control loops work and, more importantly, how they fail. As Figure 1.5 shows, a control loop can fail in three classic ways:

- **We can have no control.** We set clear expectations, such as for handwashing or for a change in our core measures, but nothing changes.

- **We can be out of control.** We think we are reducing falls, but we end up with not only more falls but also other problems. Our best-laid plans had unintended consequences.

- **We can be oscillating.** Oscillation means that we swing back and forth between two points, sometimes going out of control. An example of this might be the management team starting a program and then two months later stopping it, and then starting it up again. "Program-of-the-Month" problems often are the result of oscillations in our control loops. We keep trying different things, never sticking with one long enough to really see whether it works.

FIGURE **1.5**   Typical ways in which control loops fail

Control Loop Failure	What Happens	Potential Causes
No control	Changes in expectations do not result in any change in performance	• Data not connected to expectations • Wrong sample detail or frequency • Overmonitoring and lack of control • Poorly designed changes
Out of control	Control loop results in changes in the organization that were unexpected and unintended	• Bad data • Bad analysis • Wrong sample detail or frequency
Oscillations	Control loop sends signals to management that result in rapid swings in behavior	• Lack of data smoothing • Bad analysis

                                         Making Your Data Work

Effective data analysis and communication drives a healthy control loop.

Control loop failures are often driven by "data traps" that we need to be aware of and that we need to prevent.

Avoiding data traps: Don't collect your data at the wrong frequency

One of the first data traps is collecting data at the wrong frequency. Consider the gas gauge in your car. You sample the level of the gas tank every time you look at the gauge. Because driving the car is a "real-time" activity, you glance down at the gauge on a regular basis—probably every time you start on a journey and maybe every couple of minutes if you are getting close to running out of gas. That is probably an appropriate sampling frequency.

What if you decided that to meet your household "reporting" requirements, you needed to report on the level of the gas gauge every quarter? Is that a valid sampling frequency? Not at all! Not only is that data useless for controlling the level of gas in the tank, but the quarterly reports are also about as random as you can get—they are completely dependent on when you take the sample. If you sample the gas gauge on only a quarterly basis, you are almost guaranteed to have an event—running out of gas!

In healthcare, outside organizations often require that we report on data, sometimes on a monthly or a quarterly basis. It is vital for an organization to separate *reporting* or *monitoring* data from data used for *control* of processes.

Remember that outside organizations are using the data for a completely different purpose than you are. They are using it to monitor whether you are meeting their requirements or whether they need to intervene or even shut down your facility.

You are using the same data to control your processes to stay within the expectations you have set for your organization.

The frequency for data collection is very different for these two uses. Outside regulators can use quarterly or annual data to meet their needs, but that may not be anywhere close to the frequency you need to control your process.

An organization that tries to control a process using data that is sampled on a *monitoring* frequency is probably going to drift out of control and get into trouble. If you are using data to control your process, choose your sample frequency based on the following:

- How fast does the process normally change?

- How fast could the process go from acceptable to dangerously out of control?

- How much "early warning" do we need to get things back under control?

- What is the risk if the process goes out of control, and what is the cost to increase sampling?

There are problems with oversampling as well. Too much sampling increases costs and puts demands on resources, and if we don't produce meaningful conclusions, oversampling will result in pushback from the people who have to do the sampling.

Understand the costs associated with data collection and weigh them against the cost of the problem being addressed. Do you know the cost of each data measure that is being collected?

Collect data based on your processes' control needs, not based on a predetermined reporting schedule.

Avoid misleading conclusions caused by bad data and poor analysis

Bad data is a problem that occurs all too frequently. All data can be inherently biased, and this becomes more of a problem when it is voluntarily reported and not collected using a repeatable sampling process. Although you can use elaborate methods to design your data collection program, at a minimum, consider the following:

- Does your data represent all of the departments and functions that are involved, or is it limited to just one function, such as nursing or physicians?

- Does the collection process bias your data as being good or bad? Do you only collect exceptions, or only successes?

- Do you have a process in place to audit the collection methods and provide confidence that you understand the quality of your data?

Poor analysis is also a frequent trouble spot. Even if we collect the data effectively and are willing to accept any inherent biases, we can end up with misleading conclusions if we use poor analysis methods. Typical areas to consider include the following:

- Did we use an appropriate sample size, or are we basing our conclusions on just one or two samples?

- Do we provide some indication of what is statistically significant so we can separate the "vital few" from the "bug dust"?

- Can we confirm our conclusion using another independent analysis method or different data?

- Have we appropriately used good analysis tools such as smoothing, binning, and time series analysis?

Don't demotivate with your data

Remember that data is just part of your control loop and that the purpose of the control loop is to help you achieve your goals. Make sure that you don't accidentally demoralize your organization by the way you collect and present your data. For example, if people willingly report near-miss issues and then they feel that the data is "thrown back" in their faces, not only will the data suffer, but the whole organization will suffer as well.

Likewise, inappropriate comparisons of data between facilities within a larger system may set up competition or build conflicts that detract from achieving key goals.

Be careful of setting up metrics or goals that are self-defeating. Giving the pizza party to the group that has the best safety record for the month may result in a new employee not reporting a safety issue because he or she does not want to be the one to "ruin the run." That one decision to "not report" may offset the benefit of the entire group's efforts.

 Strive for a non-punitive data reporting process. Don't demoralize with your data.

Don't sacrifice control of your process for more monitoring

We have only a limited number of resources to collect, analyze, present, and use data. Therefore, we need to allocate them appropriately. There is constantly increasing pressure to collect additional monitoring and reporting data. Monitoring data does not change responses or outcomes; it just tells us what they are. Make sure that your organization recognizes the differences between monitoring and control data and is allocating appropriate resources to collect, analyze, and use data that will help you change behaviors and not just report on the ones that exist.

Don't present the data with the wrong level of detail

Data managers spend a lot of their time working with the data, and often they are very familiar with all the subtle variations that it includes. There is often a certain pride in the data and a desire to share the knowledge and insights that it contains. Sometimes this leads to too much of a good thing:

"If a little data is good, 20 more pages of detailed charts must be even better" is not a good assumption to make. The real value of data comes in helping people verify or change their behaviors—there really isn't much value in data for data's sake. Consider the following:

- ❑ Is the presentation useful? Does it help the user make good decisions, or is it presenting data for data's sake?

- ❑ Do we present the conclusions that have already been drawn, or do we force the end-user to try to figure out what the data means?

- ❑ Is it clear what is good data and what is bad data?

 Match your data collection, analysis, and presentation to how you plan to use the data.

Numeric data vs. exception data

The importance of exception data

If we were running a manufacturing machine that was making widgets, we could collect a large amount of parameter and specification data. We could make subtle adjustments to the control knobs on the machine and design experiments to alter the impact of all those changes. This would provide *numeric* data that would in turn enable us to control the manufacturing process to produce the largest number of high-quality widgets.

One of the key differences between manufacturing and healthcare is the degree of automation of the process. Manufacturing is often highly automated; healthcare uses some automatic pieces of equipment, but most of the processes are performed by nurses, physicians, aides, technicians, and even the patients themselves.

In comparison to much of manufacturing, healthcare has a very low level of automation. Therefore, we don't have the luxury of being able to make small adjustments on the "knobs" of the machine and tune our control loop using numeric data. Often, we must rely on *exception* data.

©2008 HCPro, Inc.

Rather than telling us a specific pressure or speed, exception data tells us when something has gone wrong—someone fell or a particular medication was late. These are exceptions to our smoothly running process (where ideally there would be no exceptions).

A good example of exception data is the occurrence report. Ideally, an occurrence report is written every time our process does not perform in the way we expect. Because we don't have a "medication knob" and a "medication digital readout" on our nursing floor like we might have a "speed knob" on a manufacturing machine, we have to rely on the exceptions to our process as data and use them as a key part of our control loop.

This leads to problems:

- The exception data often is not shared

- The exception data often has a long time lag

- The exception data requires different analysis methods to use effectively

 Share your exception data between risk management and the process control functions.

Use exception data to help control your processes

Historically, the incident or occurrence reports (exception data) were collected and managed by the Risk Management or Legal department because these reports were initially designed to deal with documenting potential litigation or potentially compensable events (PCEs). Sometimes, this led to this data being tightly protected and not shared within the hospital or healthcare facility. If this happens, it eliminates one key source of control data within the organization.

Healthcare facilities must use exception data (occurrence reports) to help control their processes.

The Risk Management and Legal departments and the performance improvement/quality/infection control functions must collectively recognize how important it is to fully use exception data to improve your processes and thereby reduce risk.

Reduce the time lag on your occurrence and incident data

If the occurrence and incident report data is to become an effective part of your control loop, you need to reduce the time lag in that data collection system. If the results from the occurrence/incident reports are not available until several months after the time of occurrence, the lag makes it very difficult to control the process. If there is no specific numeric data (i.e., no "medication digital readout") and the process relies on exception data (occurrence reports), this lag can be a significant disadvantage and can result in a significant breakdown in the control loop.

Use appropriate methods to analyze exception data

You can use many of the methods we will discuss in the following chapters to analyze exception data. A couple of key methods are particularly useful:

- Weighted significance, which we will discuss in Chapter 3

- Common cause analysis, which we will discuss in Chapter 8

CHAPTER

2

Understanding the Different Types of Data

Types of data

The more we understand the different types of data and can communicate the purposes of each to everyone from the board to the frontline staff, the more effective we will be in getting our data to benefit the organization.

In the following sections, we will look at the differences between:

- Protection, control, and monitoring data

- Outcome, problem, activity, and process data

- "What" data vs. "why" data

Protection, control, and monitoring data

You can view data in an organization as supporting one of the following three goals:

- Protecting people and physical assets

- Controlling processes

- Monitoring process health

Figure 2.1 shows how the analogy of a car on a cross-country trip (which we discussed in this book's Introduction) and the healthcare environment would correspond to these three goals.

FIGURE 2.1 Where healthcare factors fit the three goals

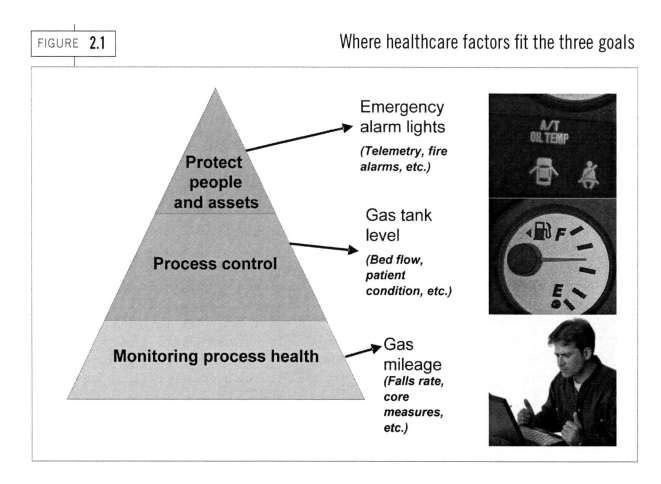

Data related to protecting people and assets

Look at the top of the pyramid in Figure 2.1. If we return to our analogy of a car on a cross-country trip, the emergency warning lights on the dashboard indicate problems such as low fuel or a hot engine in a way that is designed to cut through the clutter and that should trigger immediate responses. These pieces of data usually appear only when the people or the physical assets are in imminent danger.

In the healthcare environment, these emergency warning lights are our telemetry and life-safety alarms, and ideally, data that warns us of significant and sentinel events. But to be effective, these pieces of data must cause an immediate and appropriate response.

Data related to process control

Data used to control our processes must be a part of an effective, closed control loop. For example, to be effective in process control, bed-flow data must directly change our behaviors in a predictable way.

                                           Making Your Data Work

Remember one of the definitions of *sentinel*: "to observe the approach of danger, and give notice of it." Do you use your sentinel events as early warnings?

Likewise, when we take vital signs, they should validate our actions or change our immediate behaviors in a predictable way—if they do, then the data is part of the overall control loop.

Data related to monitoring process health

When we collect all our gas receipts at the end of the month and calculate our car's gas mileage, this is really a process monitoring task. We are not changing the control loop that tells us how hard to push down on the accelerator, nor are we changing the temperature of the engine or the speed of the car.

However, monitoring gas mileage allows us to get a very important overview function. It is a broad indicator of our car's health and our driving practices. If the gas mileage is starting to drop off, we might consider getting a tune-up or perhaps changing the procedures we use to operate the car.

Similarly, in healthcare, we monitor core measures, outcomes, fall rates, medication error rates, and a host of other measures. All of these help us to determine whether the process is healthy or whether our hospital processes need a tune-up.

Outcome, problem, activity, and process data

In addition to protecting, controlling, and monitoring data, it is also useful to subdivide data into additional categories related to outcomes, *problems*, *activities*, and *processes*, as shown in Figure 2.2.

FIGURE 2.2

Outcomes, problems, activities, and processes

Type of Data	Examples	What It Tells Us
Outcome data	• Core measures etc.	Are we delivering products and services that are meeting the expectations of the organization and the stakeholders?
Problem data	• Occurrence reports • Calibration problems • Broken equipment reports • Maintenance work orders	What are the specific exceptions that indicate times when our processes are not working as planned?
Activity data	• How many activities are on time • Critical path delays • Costs per activity • Time spent per activity	How effectively are we completing our improvement activities to address areas identified as process weaknesses?
Process data	• Throughput • Variability on the process • Trends	Is the process healthy, independent of outcomes?

"What" data vs. "why" data

Often, organizations become frustrated when their data indicates a certain trend, such as an increase in noncompliance with a particular process or procedure. We collected the data, it shows that people are not doing what we expect, and we assigned a team and gave them all the data—so why can't we fix the problem?

A key stumbling block is not recognizing that there is "what" data and "why" data. Let's look at each of these two types of data.

"What" data tells us "what is happening"

"What" data is just that: It tells us *what* is happening. "A patient fell on 5 West" is a good example of data that tells us what happened. Likewise, much of our outcome data and core measures data is "what" data. "Sixty percent of the bed heads were not elevated to the correct level" tells us what is happening on floors that have that type of bed. If that is not consistent with our expectations, we decide to change it. But therein lies the rub: We do not know enough, just from that data, to effectively change the behaviors, processes, or equipment that is causing it to happen.

Before we can effectively change our control loop for bed head elevations or any other process, we need to know *why* it is happening.

A key point to remember and constantly share with your organization is "You can't fix a 'what'—you can only fix a 'why.' "

 You can't fix a "what"; you need to create, collect, and analyze "why" data.

"Why" data tells us "why it is happening"

So where do we get "why" data? The only way to get *why* data is to do conduct analysis to determine what the cause of the problem was. This is the purpose of root cause analysis (RCA), apparent cause analysis (ACA), our improvement teams, etc. Improvement teams are sent out on missions to find out why something happened so that we can effectively address the underlying problem and change our outcomes. Figure 2.3 compares the differences between typical *what* and *why* data.

FIGURE **2.3**

"What" data versus "why" data

	Examples of "What" is happening	Examples of "Why" it is happening
Outcome data	Infection rate increased 5% last month	Noncompliance with handwashing
Problem data	Missed medications up 9% on 5 West	Lack of an effective method to handle meds when the patient is off the floor
Activity data	Redesigning the procedure is three months late	Lack of ownership of the process improvement activity

CHAPTER

3

Analysis of Your Data

Count, severity, and normalization

Before you start to analyze your data, you need to think about *count*, *severity* and *normalization*.

One of the first and simplest things we do as we start to analyze our data is to count things. We count the number of falls, or we count the number of patients that have a specific outcome. Counting events or number of outcomes is a good place to start, but there are two risks to just "counting."

The first risk in looking only at counts is that doing so can be misleading because it does not consider severity or normalization. Let's evaluate two cases.

Case 1: Severity. You are working hard to improve your medication error reduction program and have been tracking the number (*count*) of medication errors carefully for the past two years. Even though you have implemented many interventions, the total number of medication errors has not decreased significantly. You are getting frustrated.

One of the first things to look at is the *severity* of the errors. If the severity of the errors has decreased, then even though you have the same number of events reported, you are making clear progress. Remember that severity is what we want to reduce because it is directly connected to harm. The medication error count is only one part of the picture.

Always consider the severity of the event or outcomes you are counting.

Case 2: Normalization. You work in the quality group of a large system that has five hospitals. You are trying to compare performance between the facilities related to the number of obstetric outcomes. One hospital always seems to be doing exceptionally well, with only two negative outcomes reported. But this just doesn't ring true in your mind.

Whenever you compare counts or numbers of occurrences, you need to check the normalization of your data. Maybe that hospital performs only 10 deliveries each year compared to 300 at another facility. Comparing raw numbers that have not been normalized for volume would be misleading. The hospital with two bad outcomes out of 10 deliveries has a 20% negative outcome rate, whereas the hospital with 30 negative outcomes out of 300 deliveries has only a 10% negative outcome rate. That might be more useful.

Always consider the normalization of your data to adjust for differences in volume, season, acuity, and so on.

The second risk in focusing on counts is that it can reduce reporting. For example, if you present data to senior management that indicates there have been 20 falls this month (counts), and management replies with "That's unacceptable—we don't want to see that many falls reported next month," what happens? People will stop reporting the minor falls, and the numbers will look better. Then people will stop reporting the falls that are slightly more serious in nature but that aren't classified as major falls, and the numbers will look even better. Before you know it, you have significantly damaged your reporting culture, and, even worse, you have lost your stream of good data. (See the sidebar "Playing games with your indicators.")

Playing games with your indicators

Yes, it happens: People play games with your indicators and try to make themselves look good, so you need to make sure you design your methods to deal with that.

One of the benefits of looking at average severity as an overall indicator of performance in an exception reporting process is that when people start to "game" the indicator, they at least move in the right direction.

For example, let's say a Med/Surg floor is trying to reduce the average severity of its medication event reports, but then has a very serious serious event—let's say an 80-point severity event. Now, that will push up the average severity per report and the Quality Department can monitor the change. But the department members want to get the average severity back down, so they figure that if they report a larger number of smaller events, that they will bring down the average and they will look good again.

On first blush, you hate to have people try to manipulate your indicators, but look at the outcome in this case. If you were with the Quality/Performance Improvement, or Patient Safety department, following a serious event, you might counsel the department to "pay even more attention to details," "look for the little stuff," "keep your eyes open," "don't let anything slip past you," and so on.

Did you achieve that result by having the department report smaller events to get the average severity down? Absolutely! We would love to have all things be done for the right reasons, but at least it gets done and we improve!

Compare this to monitoring counts. After a serious event, the director says, "I don't want to see any more of those!" So the folks in the department become concerned about being the ones to bring up a problem and the reporting starts to drop off. Pretty soon, you have lost your control loop and things start to rapidly get worse. Just because of what you measured! Scary, isn't it?

Remember that in event reporting, you want an increasing number of reports with a decreasing severity. This is vital so that you can have confidence in your analysis of your occurrence and event reporting systems. If the number of reports is not increasing, it is almost impossible to determine whether there is a real performance improvement or whether the change is due to a reduction in reporting. The fastest solution here is to drive for constantly increasing reporting. Then you can base your decision about improvement on the change in severity. If people are reporting more medication events, but all the ones they are finding are less severe than those you have seen in the past, you are improving.

Remember, the counts tell you the number of reports and not much else. These should always be going up.

Now, what if you add the *sums* of the severities? Then you'll have some indication of the events' overall burden on the organization. Big events have a big burden, and smaller events have a smaller individual burden. But what if you have several hundred small events? They start to add up. You may see that the burden of all the small events is significantly affecting the organization's ability to perform, and it may be more damaging than the one or two isolated large events.

Another great indicator to use is the *average* severity per report. That is just the sum of the severity divided by the count. This tells you whether people are reporting bigger or smaller problems. Ideally, we would always want to see the average severity going down. As long as the counts are staying up, a decreasing average severity is a great way to demonstrate improvement in the organization. Typically, increasing counts and decreasing severity says, "We are looking harder for problems, and those that we find are not as severe as those we used to find." But you can never stop looking.

The best way to handle the count problem is to get into the habit of looking at your data through three windows. Look at:

- The number
- The weighted severity
- The average severity

Look at counts, total sum of severity, and average severity when you analyze events.

Figure 3.1 shows how to approach this data view.

FIGURE **3.1**   Counts, sum, and average

Type of Analysis	Examples	Benefits or Disadvantages
Counts	Number of falls Number of delayed medications Number of patients that get smoking cessation advice	**Benefit:** easy to use **Disadvantages:** hard to compare and leads to under-reporting
Sum of weighted severity	Total burden because of all our falls	**Benefit:** Depends on volume of reports
Average weighted severity per count	Average severity/fall Average severity/indication Average severity/near miss	**Benefits:** Adjusts for reporting volume Simple, high=level indicator Improves low=threshold reporting **Disadvantages:** Requires constant or increasing reports

Using weighted significance/severity

Providing a severity for each occurrence is very useful, especially in your analysis of occurrence reports. It is simple to do and greatly increases the value of the resulting conclusions.

Each occurrence or event report should have a significance or severity indicator that has been assigned to it. Yes, sometimes these are not accurate or updated, but let's start with what we have.

The first step is to convert each significance or severity indicator into a numerical value. Figure 3.2 provides an example of a weighting scale that converts the severity levels to a number. We will call this the *weighted severity/significance*.

FIGURE **3.2**   Typical severity rating scale

Reached patient?	Harm or no harm?	Temporary or permanent harm?	Weighting
Did not reach patient	No harm	No harm	0 – 15
Reached patient	No harm	No harm	15 – 35
Reached patient	Harm	Temporary harm	35 – 60
Reached patient	Harm	Permanent harm	60 – 80
Reached patient	Harm	Preventable death	100

The next step is to use the weighted significance. Chapter 9 covers creation and use of pivot tables in Microsoft Excel. You will use the weighted significance as a key part of your pivot table analysis.

To take full advantage of your near miss reporting, you may want to have your severity formula combine the actual severity plus the potential severity. For example, if the event reached the patient but was caught in the nick of time by someone going "above and beyond" before it could cause harm, the actual severity might be about 20 points. But this was a near miss because none of our formal processes prevented the problem. If the person hadn't "caught" it, the severity might have been permanent harm. Therefore, the potential severity might be 60.

You may add the actual and the potential severity together to give a better indication of the actual risk. (In more sophisticated settings, there might be a weighting factor to adjust the actual and potential severity.)

Develop a formal, numeric method of weighting severity.

Direction, variability, and rate

Now that you have adjusted your data for severity and you have normalized it, if appropriate, start using the data to answer a few questions so that it is useful in the control loop.

You will want to be able to evaluate and provide feedback to the organization on the following three key areas:

- Direction
- Rate
- Variability

Show all three in your data presentations.

 Direction, variability, and rate: Show all three in your data presentations.

Direction

The *direction* of a trend is a key output of your analysis. You always have to be able to answer the question "Are we getting better or worse?" That is the usually first question that your audience will ask.

In a control loop, direction is important because it helps to determine what action you should take to bring the system back under control. For example, if a room is getting colder (*direction*), you know that you need to adjust the thermostat to increase heat.

The primary way we indicate direction is through a ***trend line***. A trend line is a line that fits through our data and shows the direction. It can be a straight line or can be a curve fit, but we rely on it for the direction.

Variability

Ideally, all of your data would be nice and smooth. However, because you are measuring real-world processes—and people processes—the data often moves up and down and is rarely smooth. This volatility or variability is important because it tells you how predictable your process is and whether you can reasonably draw conclusions from your data.

A process that is highly variable will have the up and down spikes we often see: One month the value will be high, and the next month the value will be low.

Be cautious of asking your leadership to draw "direction" conclusions from highly variable data, which is often misleading. Instead, focus on the variability to indicate the predictability of the process, and then smooth the data to help you see direction.

Methods such as rolling averages or moving averages are effective to smooth highly variable data and to look for direction information within the data.

Figure 3.3 shows a highly variable data set that would be of little use to help answer the question "Are we getting better?" The raw variable data has been smoothed into a direction trend that indicates that the long-term average of the process is relatively flat, with a slight increase. You would never see that from the variable data.

Be cautious, though: If your data is too variable, it may really just be random noise—and you could be misleading your organization if you jump to conclusions from noise.

Monitor the goal's variability *and* its long-term rate of change.

FIGURE **3.3**

Monitoring variability as well as direction

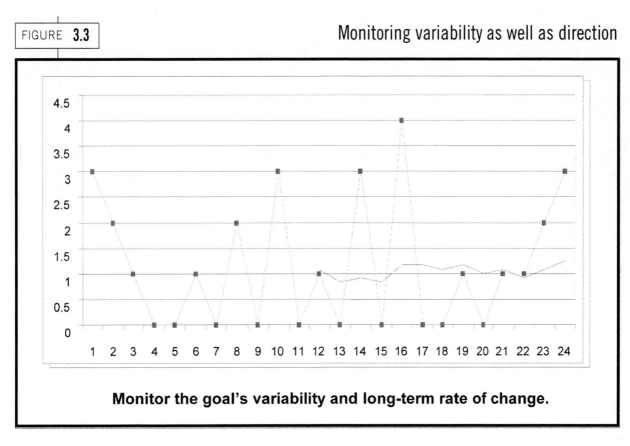

Monitor the goal's variability and long-term rate of change.

Rate

The third characteristic you are trying to pull from the data is the *rate* of change (in a chart, the rate of change is the slope of the line—the rise divided by the run). For example, if your fall reduction process data is indicating an overall reduction in the severity of falls on 7 West, the next question you need to ask is, "Are we improving fast enough, or are we not really getting much traction?"

That question is really asking what the rate of change is. If the rate of change is low, even if it is going in the right direction, you may take years to reach your goal. If the rate of change is too fast, you may lose control and not be able to sustain the change.

Two graphical methods: Binning and time series analysis

Graphical analysis of your data is a powerful tool to help you see and communicate information from what starts out as generally boring numbers. Good graphical analysis helps "mine" the information you might not see if you were looking just at the raw numbers in a list or table.

We have all made charts and graphs, and most of us are quite proficient doing so. In this section, we will discuss two graphical methods that you will use regularly to analyze your data. These two methods are *binning* and *time series analysis*.

Binning

Binning uses histograms or Pareto diagrams to compare data that you have "put into bins" to indicate what the largest contributors were over a specified period. Binning is a comparative tool that helps you make decisions about the relative contributions of the data. Figure 3.4 shows an example.

FIGURE **3.4**   Example of binning

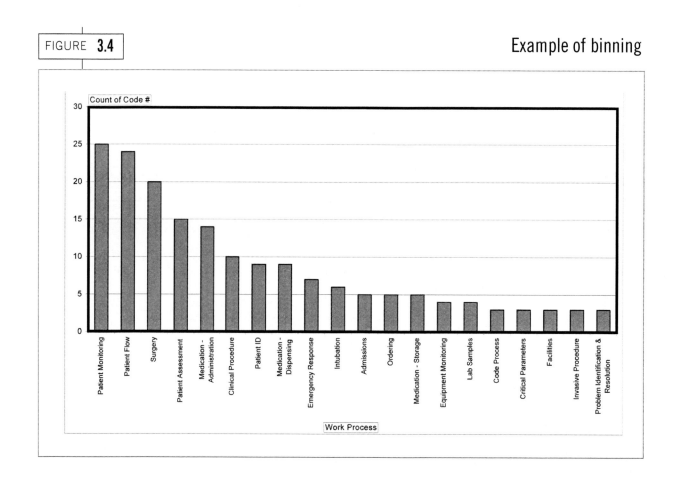

The real value of binning starts when you can look at your comparative data in multiple directions. This lets you zoom in and mine the data for a more detailed answer. For example, in Figure 3.4, we see that patient monitoring is the largest contributor in the data we are evaluating. Then, by looking at the same data using two bins (as in Figure 3.5), we can determine that misjudgments were the largest contributor to the patient monitoring events.

As long as we have useful data, we can keep adding bins to the analysis and make our diagnosis more specific.

FIGURE **3.5**   Multidimensional binning

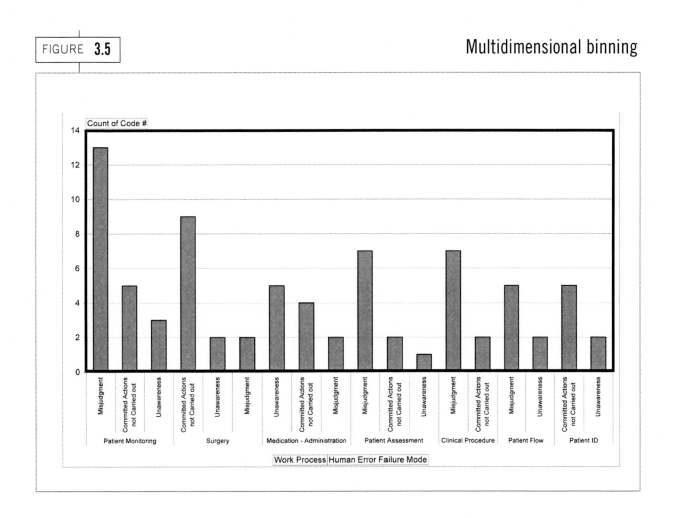

Time series analysis

A time series shows how the data changes over time and is used to help us see direction, variability, and rate. If you look back at the histograms or binning analysis, you see that there is no indication of changes over time. With a histogram, you select a period (e.g., this month, the past two years, etc.) and then look at the distribution within that period.

A time series analysis, on the other hand, looks at the changes in the data over time, as Figure 3.6 shows. This is what makes it useful when you are evaluating direction, variability, and rate, all of which are functions of time.

FIGURE **3.6**   Example of time series analysis

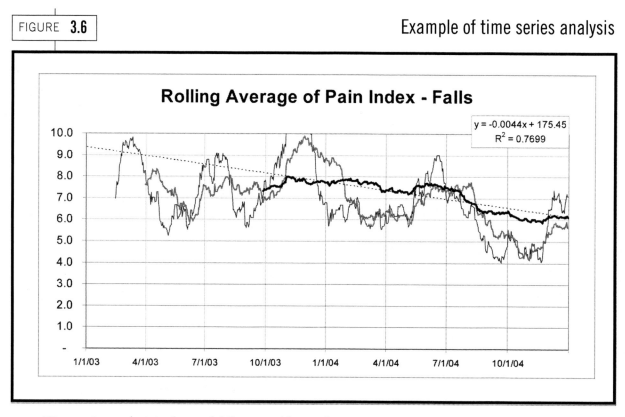

Time series analysis is also useful for two additional reasons:

- Time series analysis can provide us with a pseudo-leading indicator. If we know the direction and rate that we are going, we can make a pretty good guess as to where we will end up if we don't change anything. This is a good leading indicator of the future; however, we call it a "pseudo" leading indicator because none of us can predict the future!

FIGURE **3.7** Using time series to indicate improvement or decline

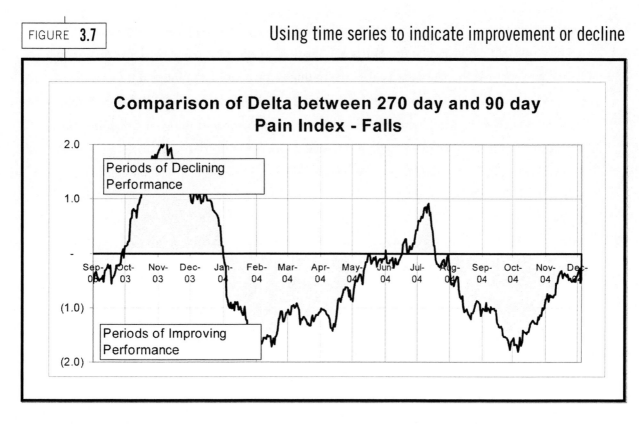

- Time series analysis is a great way to demonstrate an improvement or a decline in a process, as shown in Figure 3.7

Smoothing the data

Much of the data we use in healthcare has a high degree of variability. Sometimes this is because of variability in the process, but often it is because we don't have continuous samples.

This high degree of variability often makes it hard to determine the direction and, subsequently, to determine whether the rate of change is acceptable.

An important data analysis technique is to smooth the data to remove some of the variability and therefore help to unmask the underlying direction and rate.

In Figure 3.8, the thin line represents the raw data. It has lots of spikes and a rolling wave pattern. Trying to determine whether this is increasing or decreasing becomes difficult. The medium dark line has been smoothed by using a four-month rolling average, which just means "pick a time, average all of the data going back four months, and use this as your value." Then we move forward one step (day, week, month, etc.) and calculate the rolling average for that point, and then for the next point. This smooths the data and takes out some of the variability, as well as some of the detail.

It is still difficult to say confidently whether this line is improving, declining, or remaining flat, so we add another rolling average. This time we will use a longer average—in this case, one year. This means that every point on the chart is the average of the past year's values. Then we move forward one step and do it again.

Notice that with the one year moving average, almost all of the higher-frequency variability has been removed, leaving a clearer underlying trend—in this case, sloping down at a moderate rate.

FIGURE 3.8

Smoothing your data with rolling averages

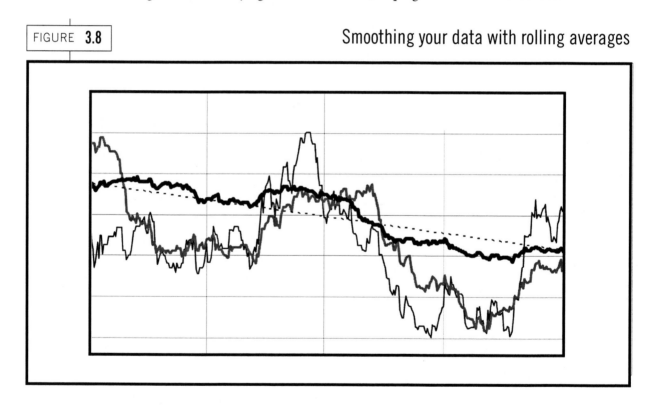

 Always smooth your data to remove the variability before you try to determine direction or rate.

The use of rolling or moving averages is a very useful technique to smooth your data. It also lets you use a technique called crossing averages, explained further in Chapter 5.

Other analysis methods

Data analysis is a very well-developed science and can become deeply complex. Methods and techniques to help you get additional value from your data are constantly being developed.

Our objective in this book is to give you the tools and techniques you will use every day to deliver effective analysis to your organization. Remember that a wealth of more complex statistical tools and methods, such as Six Sigma and advanced statistics, are available to help you to use your data to assist in making decisions.

Before you invest your own or your organization's time or energy into more sophisticated methods, however, it is beneficial to become familiar and comfortable with the simple hammer and screwdriver tools presented here. We have selected the simple tools that you will be using every day when you analyze or present data. Learn them well, and then add the more complex tools when you have a specific need for them.

> Start simple with your analysis techniques, and build up to more sophisticated methods such as Six Sigma and advanced statistics.

CHAPTER

4

Data Coding: If It's Not in a Bin, You Will Never Find It

Integrating coding with your protection, control, and monitoring programs

To successfully use the techniques we have discussed so far, you need to first:

- Be able to find the data you are looking for

- Look at it from different perspectives

Coding is the process we use to identify data so that we can find it and look at it effectively.

Some organizations go overboard when coding their data, which can result in a large expenditure of resources. Conversely, some organizations collect data and assume that the "gold" will jump out at them without having to do any coding. Others code the right volume, but they don't get the results they would like because they haven't thought through the codes and bin structure thoroughly enough.

Coding should serve your needs and directly support your programs. A good test is to ask the following question regarding each piece of coding you ask for on a form or enter into your database: "If that particular code/bin pops up in a trend, will we know what to do to improve our overall performance?"

Know what you would do if a particular code group jumps out in a trend. The starting point is a well-designed code structure.

The importance of a good coding structure

When you collect exception data, you immediately code it. This coding process puts the data into bins—bins for medication errors, falls, delays, and so on. Likewise, outcome data is collected in bins for all the core measures. We code data by demographic information (age, sex, floor, weight, etc.), and that puts the data into bins. Putting data into bins is a natural way for us to compare data.

The success of your *histogram* or *binning analysis* really starts with your selection of bins. Unfortunately, we often inherit bins left over from a previous data collection form or bins that are constrained because we "can't change the software." That can make our job harder.

If we had complete control over the bins in which we collect our data, how would we design them? A well-designed coding structure should result in bins that:

- Are the correct size

- Are easily rolled up

- Can be looked at cross functionally

- Are consistently applied

Figure 4.1 summarizes the guidelines for bin structure.

FIGURE **4.1**

Guidelines for the design of codes and bins

Bins must not be too big	If the bin is too big, you will collect too many samples in that bin and lose resolution in your analysis. If you see that one bin has 40% to 50% of your samples in it, you may want to consider splitting that into smaller bins.
Bins must not be too small	If you have too many bins, the number of pieces of data that show up in each bin goes down and you may not see a clear "top contributor." If you have a large number of bins with only one or two samples in each, think about combining them. If your histogram is flat and does not clearly indicate a group of major contributors, you may have too many bins.
Make sure that your binning codes can be rolled up	Your data needs to serve different people, and this means you may need different levels of detail. Make sure that your binning codes can be rolled up. For example, you might like your "Medication delays because patient was off the floor" data to roll up into the "Medication Delays" bin, which you would like to roll up into all of the "Medication Errors" bins, which might roll up into the "Clinical Errors" bin. Remember that binning codes can roll up into different totals. Design that into your binning code structure.
Make sure that the coding is consistent	Make sure that your interpretation and definition of the bins are consistent. If one person is responsible for all the coding, that should happen naturally. If you have everyone who submits an event report code their own data, you need to make sure that the definitions of the bins are clear; otherwise, different people will but things in different places.
Multiple attributes	Binning is used to diagnose and trigger activities on the largest contributors. Make sure that you have different bins for different attributes. For example, for exception data, you will want a bin for where the problem occurred, a different bin for when it occurred (during what shift), and another bin for the process that was being used. Be careful that you do not mix different attributes in the same bin.

FIGURE **4.1**

Guidelines for the design of codes and bins (cont.)

Be careful of yes/no coding	Sometimes your data collection software provides a field with a yes/no answer or a box that is checked. When you are binning data you are interested in comparisons, so yes/no bins are of limited use. For example, a bin that is labeled "Bed Rails Up?" and expects a yes or no answer will not be as useful as a bin labeled "Bed Rail Position" and that allows a choice of "Down," "Up 1," "Up 2," "Fully Up," and "Split." It will be much easier to analyze falls with multiple values than with yes/no data.
Include demographic, "what," and "why" bins	Make sure that you have binning codes for demographic information (sex, date, time, shift, age, floor, etc.); "what" information (fall, medication, AMI, no aspirin, etc.); and "why" information (missing step in procedure, lack of experience, poor handoff, etc.).

Rolling up and down through the code structure

Your data will serve different people, and this means that you may need different levels of detail. Make sure that your binning codes can be rolled up. For example, you might like your "medication delays because patient was off the floor" data to roll up into a bin labeled "Medication Delays," which you would like to roll up into a bin labeled "All Medication Errors," which might roll up into a bin labeled "Clinical Errors."

Remember that binning codes can roll up into several different totals. Design that into your binning code structure.

The opposite of rolling up your data is being able to zoom in on it. If you present a high-level rollup of data at the executive level and they ask a question regarding the data, you want to be able to "zoom in" on the data that supports the rollup.

Make sure your coding structure allows you to roll up and roll down.

Coding traps

Your coding can also trap you and make your job harder. Some of the key coding traps include "yes/no codes," "single value vs. multiple values," and "mixing categories." Let's look at examples of these coding traps.

Example 1: Yes/no codes

Sometimes our data collection software provides a field with a yes/no answer or a box that is checked. When you are binning data, you are interested in comparisons, so yes/no bins are of limited use. For example, a bin that is labeled "Bed Rails Up?" and expects a yes/no answer will not be as useful as a bin that is labeled "Bed Rail Position" and allows a choice of "Down," "Up 1," "Up 2," "Fully Up," and "Split." It will be much easier to analyze falls with the multiple values rather than with the yes/no data.

Example 2: Mixing categories

A code set on a form might include a pull-down menu from which you can select only one answer. For example, say that a pull-down menu includes selections for "ICU Patient" and "Contact Precautions." This code set is poorly designed because those two answers are not really related, and both might be true. A better code set would have two separate fields so that the first can indicate where the patient is being treated and the second can indicate special precautions.

Example 3: Multiple values

In the preceding example, if there was a special precautions code, we might need to be able to select more than one answer. Although databases can handle multiple values in a code field, be aware that the complexity of your analysis goes up significantly when there are multiple values. It is a good practice to start by trying to have meaningful, related, single values. Sometimes allowing multiple values can cause the code set to begin to get "fuzzy," which obscures the underlying value of your data.

The *Clue* test: Can you tell a story?

You may have played the popular board game *Clue*. In the game, players are asked to solve a murder that requires them to specify who committed the murder, where, and with what weapon. This results in answers such as "Colonel Mustard in the dining room with the candlestick." The players put together data, and they slice and dice the problem until they come up with a solution in these three dimensions (which are really code categories!).

A good test for your code structure is to see whether you can tell a story just by using code categories.

For example, the code categories for your occurrence report process might result in the following: "While the [PERFORMER] who works in [DEPARTMENT] was doing [KEY ACTIVITY] in the [WORK PROCESS] using [EQUIPMENT], an [EVENT] occurred, which affected [RE-CIPIENT]. This event appears to have been caused/was caused by [CAUSE], which resulted in [CONSEQUENCE]."

To be able to tell this story and all the variations that happen for events every day, we would need to collect and code those key nine categories.

 If you can tell a story with your codes, they will probably help answer your questions.

CHAPTER

5

Comparing Your Data

Comparing your data to your goals

Once we have collected and started to analyze our data, we are often called upon by departments, senior leadership, or even the board of directors to make a "judgment call" about the results of this analysis: "Is that OK?" However, such judgment calls are really answering the question, "How do we compare to some standard?"

When we were discussing the control loop for an electric blanket in Chapter 1, you compared the measured data against a setpoint and, depending on the results of that comparison, you made appropriate adjustments. You do the same things with organizational data. You decide what corrections to make in your processes or behaviors based on how your data compares to a standard.

In our organization, the setpoints are defined by our goals. Some of these goals are big strategic targets and some are day-to-day operational targets. Remember, data needs to be part of our control loop, so we need to set clear expectations or goals to which to compare the data. Otherwise, the control loop is broken.

Types of goals

Because expectations and goals are such an important part of an effective control loop, it is important that we understand the different types of goals an organization might have. In doing so, we need to ask the question, "Are we working to meet our own goals or only to meet external requirements?"

External and internal goals

Typically, the first breakdown of goals is into *external* and *internal* goals or expectations. Targets set by The Joint Commission or by federal or state regulators are external goals. In contrast, goals that are set by the board, senior leadership, or departments are internal goals. Although you have to meet all the required goals, it is important that you "run your own ship" and that you recognize and live up to your own internal goals, not just those which are imposed upon your facility from the outside.

Organizations that try to meet only external requirements often feel overwhelmed and out of control—which can lead to poor performance because the organization has not accepted the goals as its own.

Make sure that your organization clearly sets its own internal goals and is not trying to meet only external requirements

Goals translate drivers into action. Set your own internal goals—don't just rely on external goals.

As Figure 5.1 shows, organizational goals can be divided into three main types:

- "Rallying cry" goals

- Outcome goals

- Activity completion goals

 Making Your Data Work

FIGURE **5.1**   Types of goals

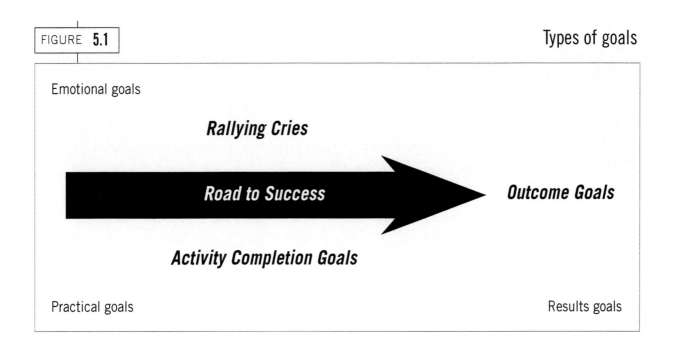

Rallying cry goals

Rallying cry goals are emotionally stirring, motivating goals that "rally the troops" and get all of us moving in the same direction. By their nature, these goals are not easily measured, but they are vitally important (see Figure 5.2).

FIGURE **5.2**   Rallying cry goals

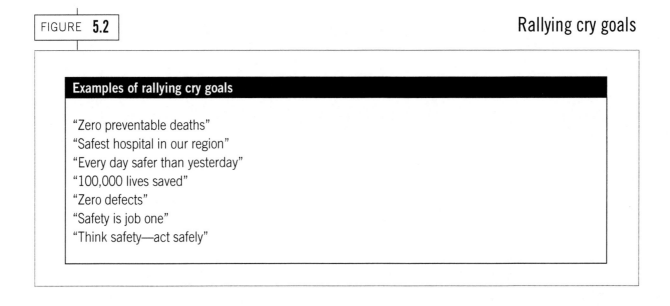

Don't limit your rallying cry goals to things you can measure.

Although rallying cry goals are essential, they do have a downside. A rallying cry goal that is selected poorly can be a demotivator when it is not reached. For example, an organizational goal to reach "Zero Preventable Deaths" is a great goal with a strong moral basis, but even if you can achieve it, you need to be cautious of overconfidence and complacency—and you need to think of the emotional impact on the organization three years later when a random, preventable death occurs. Does that mean that all of the efforts have failed? The organization must be able to deal with that.

Consider the implications of the selection of the rallying cry goal on the regulatory process as well. Achieving the overall goal and then backsliding can result in increased regulatory attention and concerns.

Even with these cautions, rallying cry goals are a key part of the expectation-setting part of the control loop.

 Be cautious of rallying cry goals that can backfire and demotivate.

Activity completion goals

Activity completion goals are all the goals we set to get things done. They are directly related to ongoing tasks and are usually easily measured. All corrective actions that come from the cause analysis process must be tracked, and we need to be able to compare the data we collect regarding their completion with our overall goals.

Comparing the activity completion data to the goals is a key part of the project management cycle and is often a major challenge in healthcare. The organization sets clear construction activity goals when building a new patient wing or a new parking structure, because we know that if we don't compare our progress data with our goals, the building will never get completed on time. We need to do the same thing with all of the organization's performance improvement activities.

Measuring activity completion goals is a critical part of the implementation step in the control loop. (See Figure 5.3.)

| FIGURE **5.3** | Examples of activity completion goals |

Activity Completion Goals

"100% of care providers trained"
"10 key processes evaluated and simplified"
"All root cause analyses completed within 45 days"
"95% of all approved performance improvement
projects completed on time"

Remember, activity goals do not indicate success in changing outcomes—they just indicate that you did what you planned.

Activity completion metrics

The science of project management specializes in measuring the process of completing activities on budget. Technology and tools are available to begin applying project management technology to healthcare activity management.

If your organization is just getting started in project tracking activities, you may want to consider the following types of metrics:

- Top 10 latest projects/activities ("List of Shame")

- Aging, or the number of days left in the schedule or the number of days late

- Percentage of all projects/activities that are completed on time

- Percentage of work on the project/activity that has been completed

Outcome goals

The last key type of goal that we use in our control loops is the type that measures outcomes. These are our quality goals and often our productivity goals. When we talk about core measures, we are talking about *outcome goals*.

Typically, outcome goals are continuous numeric measures that we compare to a standard to determine whether they are acceptable in quality, productivity, or cost.

When you set performance improvement targets, they are usually related to some outcome measure, and how you word and set these goals will determine not only what you achieve but also how the organization responds to the new target (see Figure 5.4).

FIGURE **5.4**   Examples of outcome goals

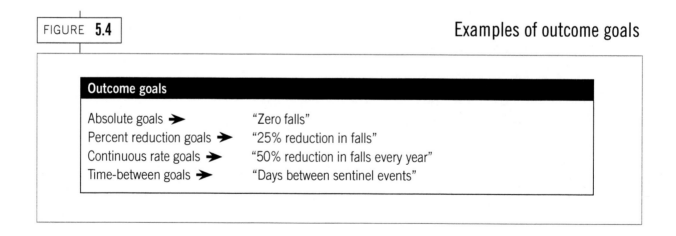

Outcome goals	
Absolute goals ➤	"Zero falls"
Percent reduction goals ➤	"25% reduction in falls"
Continuous rate goals ➤	"50% reduction in falls every year"
Time-between goals ➤	"Days between sentinel events"

Outcome goals are usually worded as either "one-time" or "continuous improvement" goals.

One-time vs. continuous improvement goals

One-time goals are worded as an absolute result, such as "Reduce falls to zero." By contrast, a *continuous improvement goal* is worded as "Reduce falls by 50% each quarter. "There are some important differences between these two methods (see Figure 5.5). A one-time goal can be demotivating because as soon as the organization stretches to reach this new goal, you raise the bar and give the organization a new, harder-to-reach goal. That can be frustrating and can result in pushback from your management and the frontline staff.

A continuous improvement goal can go on forever. If you want to make a 50% reduction in falls each quarter, in the second quarter your goal is to reduce falls to 50% of your original baseline; in the third quarter, to reduce them to 25% (a 50% reduction); in the fourth quarter, to reduce them to 12.5% (another 50% reduction); then to 6.25%; and on and on. You don't have to go back and "raise the bar," because everyone knows you expect continuous improvement.

The other key difference is that a one-time goal manages the endpoint, whereas a continuous improvement goal manages the rate of change. (Remember that one of the key trend areas is the rate.)

FIGURE **5.5** One-time goals vs. continuous outcome improvement goals

One-time goals	Continuous goals
Single improvement activity	Culture of continuous improvement
Measure the absolute results of key indicators	Measure the rate of change for key indicators
Have to "raise the bar" when goal is met	"Keep on going"
Manage the endpoint	Manage the rate of change

Examples of goal setting

Example 1: If we set a one-time goal of "90% of all medications will be delivered within 30 minutes of the scheduled time," we are focused on the endpoint of 90%. When we get there, we will have to either live with that and assume that we never have to do better, or raise the bar. In this case, we would monitor the number of late medications to provide feedback to the control loop.

Example 2: If we set a continuous improvement goal of "50% improvement in the number of medications delivered within 30 minutes of the scheduled time every ___ month," we are focused on an improvement rate. We can adjust the rate by inserting the appropriate time period in the blank. A slower rate would be a 50% reduction every 12 months. A very fast rate would be a 50% improvement every two months. You, your leadership, or the board would set the rate based on the risk, the strategy, and the capabilities of the organization. In this case, you would monitor the rate of improvement to provide feedback to the control loop.

"Compared to . . .": Setting effective targets and goals

Building on our understanding of the different types of goals, how can you design a good goal for a major process such as the patient safety process? Do you want a rallying cry goal or an outcome goal? The ideal solution may include both.

Figure 5.6 demonstrates how we can combine two types of goals to achieve an emotional rallying cry (no preventable deaths; who can argue with that?), but in a measurable, continuous fashion that would be less likely to demotivate.

 Have an emotional rallying cry goal, but demonstrate it by measurable, continuous, rate-based goals.

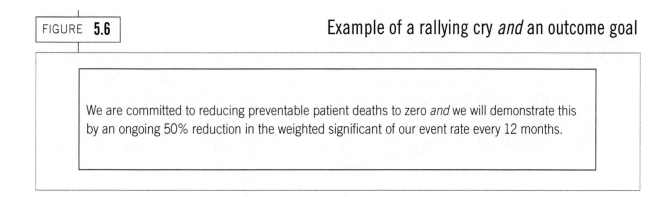

FIGURE **5.6** Example of a rallying cry *and* an outcome goal

We are committed to reducing preventable patient deaths to zero *and* we will demonstrate this by an ongoing 50% reduction in the weighted significant of our event rate every 12 months.

Using crossing averages: Comparing against ourselves

Ideally, we would like to be able to compare our performance data to that of others. We do that with benchmarks whenever possible. Unfortunately, with much of our data, there is not a clear benchmark, or there is such a large potential difference between how we measure a value and how another facility might measure the same value that the comparison is meaningless. However, that doesn't lessen the desire to compare.

A method called *crossing averages* is a very useful comparison tool. Crossing averages:

- Allows you to benchmark or compare your own performance to yourself

- Compares short-term performance to long-term performance

Figure 5.7 shows an example of crossing averages in action. The dark line is the long term (12-month) moving average, and we are comparing our short-term performance to the long-term demonstrated performance. This allows us to identify periods when we are "doing better than we used to do" (periods of improvement) and periods when we are "doing worse than we used to do" (periods of decline).

FIGURE **5.7**

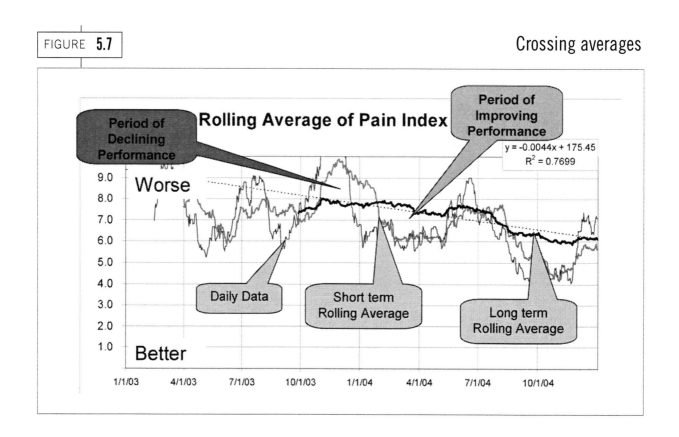

Rolling Average of Pain Index

Period of Declining Performance

Period of Improving Performance

$y = -0.0044x + 175.45$
$R^2 = 0.7699$

Worse

9.0
8.0
7.0
6.0
5.0
4.0
3.0
2.0
1.0

Better

Daily Data

Short term Rolling Average

Long term Rolling Average

1/1/03   4/1/03   7/1/03   10/1/03   1/1/04   4/1/04   7/1/04   10/1/04

Use crossing averages to compare short-term performance to long-term performance.

This is useful to indicate improvement or decline.

CHAPTER

6

Control Charts

Is the process under control?

In earlier chapters, we established the important role that data provides in the control of a system. The data helps us determine whether the process is "under control" and whether it is performing as we expected.

In the manufacturing world, the control loop for a machine that produces widgets is vitally important. If the widgets being produced are too small or too big, they will not pass inspection and instead will become scrap. We want to do everything we can to adjust the "knobs and dials" on the manufacturing machine to reliably (*every time*) produce acceptable widgets.

In manufacturing, we would monitor the data that is collected as we inspect the widgets to determine whether the machine (process) is under control.

In healthcare, we also want to know whether our processes are under control. A good tool to help monitor whether our processes are "under control" is the ***control chart***.

What is a control chart?

A control chart is simply a time series chart—sometimes called a run chart—that shows how the data points from our production "run" deviate from the specification, mean or center point. If the process is starting to produce widgets that are too big, we make a few adjustments to reduce the size and bring the process back under control.

Key parts of the control chart are:

- The plot of the actual sampled data

- A centerline of either the specification, mean, or the desired set point

- An *upper control limit* or UCL (if it gets bigger than this, we are concerned)

- A *lower control limit* or LCL (if it gets smaller than this, we are concerned)

A control chart is based on the statistical process control concept: Although there will always be some variation in the data, as long as the variation is within limits and does not show a trend, we can assume that our process is under control.

Figure 6.1 shows what a normal process that is under control might look like. Notice that none of the data points have exceeded the control limits and that there does not appear to be a trend on either side of the center line.

| FIGURE **6.1** | Control chart with a process that is in control |

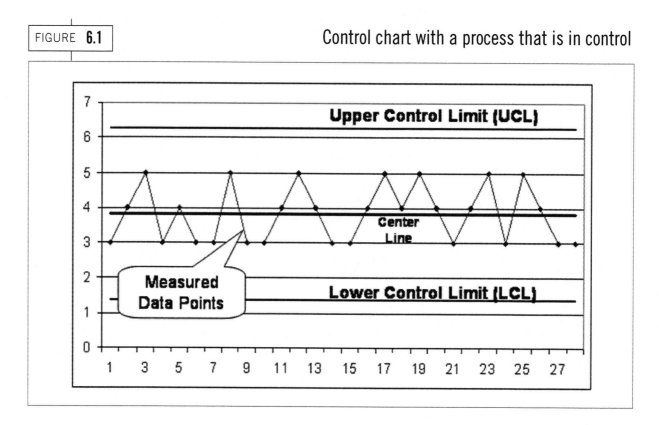

We have selected the UCL and LCL as the "guardrails" on our process. If we hit them, we know something may be wrong. Figure 6.2 shows a control chart in which one point has exceeded the UCL. That would be of interest because at that point in time, the process was not under control—something happened. If it happened once, it could happen again if we do not investigate, understand what the underlying cause was, and then adjust our process so that we are confident that it is under control. Because only a single point has gone over the UCL, we will be looking for a special kind of cause, such as a bad measurement, a one-time human error, or a situation that our process does not usually cover.

FIGURE **6.2**   Control chart with value exceeding UCL

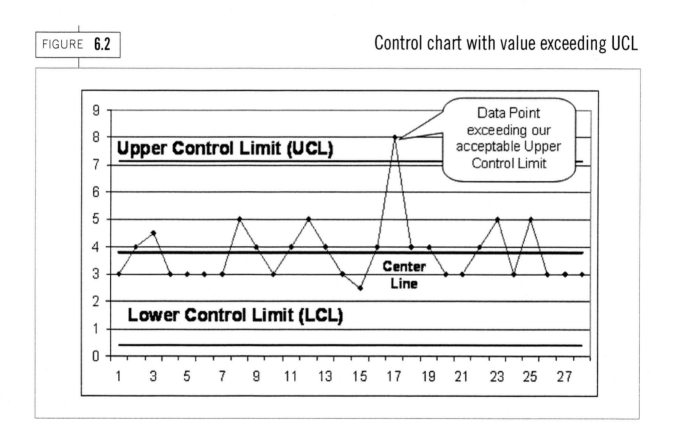

Sometimes the process starts to drift and begins to lose control in a slower fashion. We start to see values that are still within our control limits but that seem to be trending in a direction we are not happy with. This is our early warning of potential future problems. In contrast to the one single point that popped over the control limit, something different is going on here. We need to look for things that could lead to a degradation of our process. These are going to be underlying issues that are common to multiple data points rather than very specific (special) to one data point. Figure 6.3 shows the beginning of a trend, all on one side of the center line, which may be indicating an important change in the process.

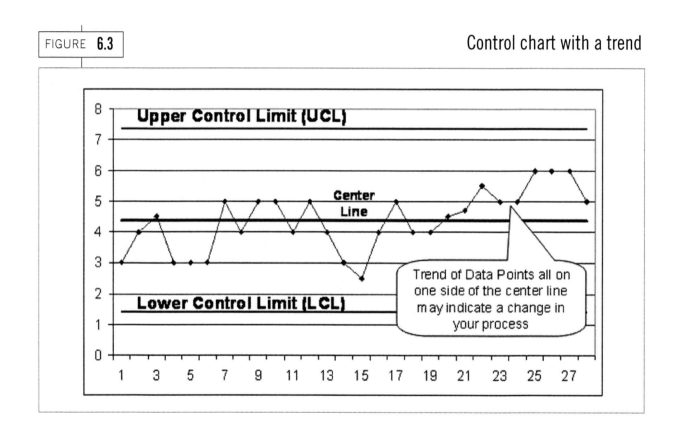

FIGURE **6.3**   Control chart with a trend

Control limits vs. specification limits

Remember that simple control charts such as those we have already discussed can help you to monitor variability and determine whether the process is under control—in other words, whether the results are repeatable.

However, repeatedly making widgets within a tight control band does not mean that you are creating *good* widgets. Make sure that your process is delivering within your *specification limits* as well.

For example, if your process repeatedly provides aspirin to a heart attack patient within 26 hours of arrival, and there is a very small deviation from 26 hours, that would indicate that your process is repeatable and, arguably, under control. Unfortunately, it does not meet the "specification limits" that require heart attack patients to have aspirin delivered within 24 hours of their arrival. You need to clearly indicate the goal or specification limit on the control chart to show that, although the process is under control, it may be out of adjustment.

If all this is making you wonder how elaborate your control chart should be, see the following short sidebar.

How Sophisticated Should We Be?

The science of statistical process control is well developed and can be quite complex. If you are going to use control charts, start with the simple understanding of what they are trying to do for you—assist in determining whether your process is within control.

In statistical process control, there are many types of control charts and much guidance on how to set control limits and monitor for trends. Don't get overwhelmed! The concept is simple, and you don't need to make it too complex.

For more information, conduct a Web search on "statistical process control" or "control charts."

Setting the control limits

Setting the control limits (UCL and LCL) is an important part of analyzing your data using control charts. Think of the UCL and the LCL as "guardrails with alarms" that sound to alert you to problems. You want to make sure that they tell you in enough time, but you don't want a lot of false alarms.

You can set your UCL and LCL in two main ways:

1. You decide—control limits are based on your requirements for the process

2. Statistically—usually based on the number of *standard deviations* above or below your center point

If you are not certain about where you want to set your UCL and your LCL, a good starting point is to just draw lines at one standard deviation, two standard deviations, and three standard deviations. Typically, three standard deviations is used as an indication of a process being "out of control," Three standard deviations was selected as a compromise between giving a good alert and reducing false alarms.

If you draw multiple control limit lines—as shown in Figure 6.4—you can watch as the data moves between them, allowing you to decide whether a data point that crosses one of the lines is an *alert* point.

FIGURE **6.4**   Control charts with standard deviation bands

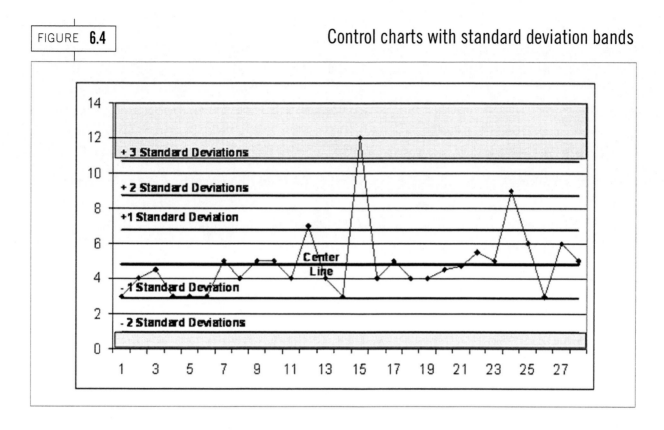

If your process is staying within the one-standard-deviation bands, it is relatively tightly controlled. Exceeding the three-standard-deviation bands indicates a loss of process control, and exceeding the two-standard-deviation bands indicates an area to watch.

So, how do you calculate the standard deviations? The theory is available in many introductory books on statistics, but in reality, you will use a function in Excel or equivalent software to calculate them, or you'll buy statistical process control software to add onto Excel.

Not all data works in control chart form. Control charts, like all analysis methods, are tools in your toolbox and are not the only way to see whether your processes are in control.

Make sure that you know how control charts will be useful to your organization before you invest a lot of money and time in them!

Control chart traps

Control charts are not always the easiest choice for an analysis technique. For example, say you want to determine whether your aspirin process is under control. First, you need to determine what type of data to collect. You have three choices:

- Percentage of patients that get aspirin within 24 hours (this would be the percent acceptable)

- Percentage of patients that do not get aspirin within 24 hours (this would be the percent defective, which is often called a P-chart)

- Average length of time to provide aspirin (parameter value)

You also know that there is an upper specification limit of 24 hours (1,440 minutes). Now you need to determine whether a control chart is the best tool. Often, we see charts that show percentage of compliance. Figure 6.5 shows the percentage of patients that get aspirin.

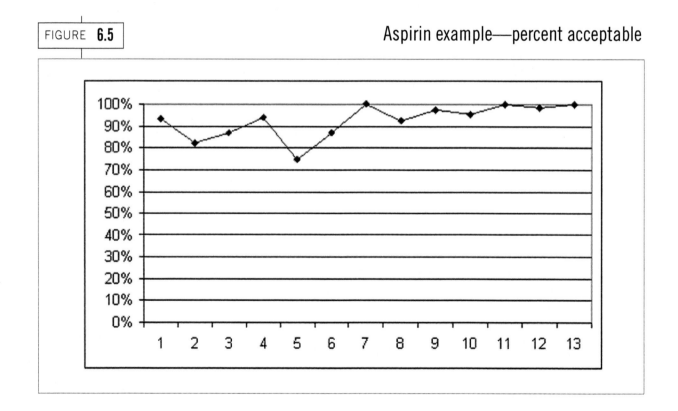

FIGURE **6.5**   Aspirin example—percent acceptable

©2008 HCPro, Inc.   **Making Your Data Work**

Don't trap yourself without a way to improve your performance!

Because this is a goal, we are often tempted to display our data in this way. When we share this data, most people will say, "Great! It looks like we are meeting our goals. Maybe we can move a little energy to another project."

One of the problems of plotting "percent acceptable" is that when you get close to 100%, it all starts to blend together. Then you have backed your continuous improvement philosophy into a corner with no place to go—except to another project.

In this case, would it make sense to put the UCL and LCL on the chart? Not really. We are not interested in setting a center line as a goal—we can't get above 100%. And there really is not much "acceptable space" below the line, so the LCL would not make sense. Therefore, this is better presented as a trend rather than a control chart.

We can turn this over and present the data as the number of defects, or the number of times a person did not get aspirin within the time limit. In the control chart world, this would be called a P-chart (see Figure 6.6).

FIGURE **6.6**

Example of a P-chart

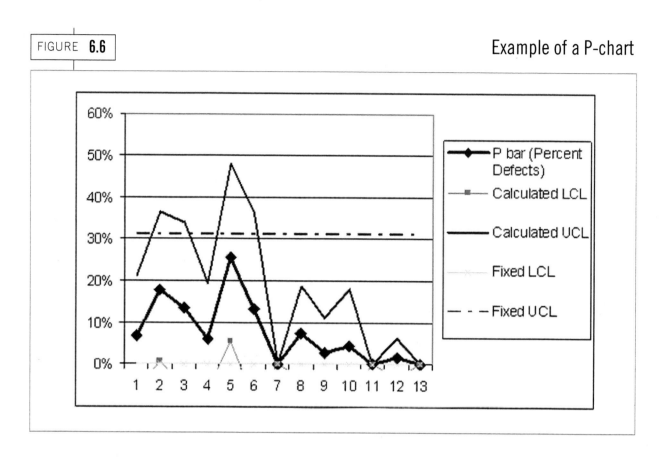

Now we can either select a fixed control limit to alert us to a change in the process or we can recalculate the control limits for each month. If we use a fixed control limit, that makes it easy but does not encourage improvement. Conversely, if we recalculate the control limits every month, poor performance may become the norm.

You can be more sophisticated and use a moving average for the control limits to make them smoother and more realistic.

Make sure that you understand why you are putting control limits on your graphs and where they come from.

Now, instead of looking at the percentage that is unacceptable (defects) or the percentage that is acceptable, let's look at just the average time to get aspirin into each patient. Figure 6.7 takes a modified approach: It plots the average time to deliver aspirin to a heart attack patient, and the graph compares that average to our previous long-term average (in the figure, the historical center line is 480 minutes) when we thought things were going well. Instead of a UCL, in this case we use the specification limit (i.e., aspirin must be given to heart attack patients less than 24 hours after admission). We also smooth out the data so that we see the bigger picture as well as the monthly variations.

When we look at the data in this way, we get a completely different story!

| FIGURE **6.7** | Comparison of aspirin delivery; average to previous long-term average |

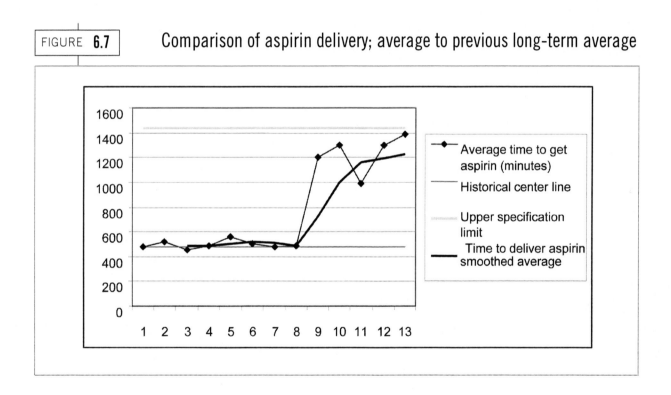

Maybe we aren't really getting better. It looks like there have been some long delays for some patients, and those incidents are really moving our "time to deliver" up. In fact, as a process, we are getting very close to having all of our patients slip over into "Unacceptable." Something must have happened. We need to investigate quickly because we are only a month or so away from crossing the 24-hour line for the average.

The message? Use control charts and all the analysis tools as part of an overall, thorough, and credible analysis. One tool may not tell the whole story. (See Figure 6.8.)

When building control charts, pay close attention to your sampling frequency. If your sample is not large enough or continuous enough, your data may be misleading.

| FIGURE **6.8** | Suggested rules to determine alerts and trends on control charts |

- One or more points outside the UCL or LCL or three standard deviation lines.
- Two or three consecutive points outside the two standard deviation lines.
- Four or five points consecutively outside the one standard deviation line.
- Seven to nine points all on the same side of the center line may be an important early warning of a trend, even if they have not crossed any of your limit lines.

Making control charts

Follow these step-by-step instructions to make an effective control chart:

1. Decide whether you are going to control the process by monitoring the number of defects (P-chart) or by monitoring a variable or parameter (time to deliver, etc.).

2. Make sure that you have adequate data. One or two points won't help much.

3. Plot the data in time.

4. Determine the upper and lower alert and control limits.

5. Calculate them based on standard deviations, use predetermined specification limits, or select them using other methods.

6. Interpret the chart. Determine what the data is telling you.

7. Look for points outside the control limits.

8. Look for trends (big and small).

9. Analyze why the process is moving out of control.

10. Determine what corrective actions you will take to get it back on track.

11. Cause changes!

CHAPTER

7

Trending: Listening to Your Data

Why do we trend?

If data is there to serve us, we need to listen to it as we would a wise advisor—and we need to pay attention when it speaks to us. In a very practical way, trends are how our data speaks to us. Organizations that have good trend programs "hear" lots of interesting things from their data. In organizations that do not effectively trend, data is "silent," and staff members wonder why they don't know what is going on.

A good trending program provides at least three major benefits:

- The trend process allows us to identify issues we would not have seen otherwise

- Trending provides early warnings of emerging problems

- Trending provides a high-level indicator of risk, performance, and improvement

So, what makes a good trend program? First, you need to collect and manage the right data, then you must effectively analyze the data, and finally you have to communicate it back to the organization so that changes will be made. As in so many other parts of the improvement process, the organization does not get partial credit for a great trend analysis if it does not cause change!

You invest a lot of time and effort collecting data. Are you getting real value from your trend program?

Trending is a "triggering process," not a "diagnostic process"

One of the first traps in trending is not recognizing that trending is really a "triggering" activity and not a diagnostic activity.

Trending is one of our most powerful tools for dealing with large volumes of "what" data to help us trigger other activities to further investigate the "whys" behind the trend. You must think of your trending program as a triggering activity and not as a diagnostic activity.

One of the problems that organizations have with trending is that they unrealistically develop expectations that a trend graph will automatically get to the root of the problem, as in the following example.

Example: An increase in falls

Your trend analysis shows a significant increase in falls. You present this analysis to the chief nursing officer (CNO), who appreciates the heads-up. But within moments, you are asked, "What do I do about it? This data isn't really very useful."

Your CNO has rapidly moved from the triggering ("what") world to the diagnostic ("why") world. He or she is expecting the trend tools to provide diagnostic information, which the initial trends can rarely do.

This doesn't mean the data is useless: The trends have achieved their purpose of triggering the need for some additional action—perhaps the formation of a team or implementation of a cause analysis to get to the underlying "why" questions.

 Trending causes us to "trigger" a **diagnostic** activity, which leads to a **correction** activity. *Think of trending as triggering, not diagnosing.*

 Making Your Data Work

A data-focused activity

Trending is a data-focused activity, as opposed to an event-focused activity such as failure modes and effects analysis (FMEA) or root cause analysis (RCA). An RCA typically looks at a single event that has already happened, and an FMEA looks at events that have not yet happened. [1] Trending is focused on looking at a relatively large volume of data samples and looking for meaning from them.

By definition, trends are part of the time series analysis family because they look at changes over time. When we conduct trending, we are really looking for the changes over time of the three characteristics of our data: *direction, variability*, and *rate*.

Trends look at how the direction, variability, and rate change over time.

How effective is your trend program?

Like the RCA or FMEA process, we need to monitor the effectiveness of our trend process. But how can we tell whether our trend process is healthy?

One of the key measures of the effectiveness of any trend program is the number of new issues that it triggers. If the goal of the trend program is to listen to the data, we need to know whether we are paying attention and whether the conversation is useful to us.

If your trend program doesn't usually identify anything you didn't already know, you are probably not getting real value out of all those charts and graphs. Likewise, if you can't answer how many new issues or insights your trend program has generated, an important and expensive program is being under-monitored.

One effective method to track the effectiveness of your trend program is to tag new issues. Every time the trend program identifies a new issue, enter it in your Occurrence or Incident Reporting System as an occurrence report with a CODE = TREND. Then it will be tracked and monitored, and you can prioritize the trend-triggered actions.

At the end of the year, if you see that there are only 5 or 10 insights or new issues, you have a good indication that the trend process may not be pulling its own weight.

 If you can't identify the number of actions the trend program has triggered, it probably isn't working well.

Smoothing

If the variability of the data is large, it often can mask the underlying *direction* of the data. And if we can't see the underlying direction, it is very difficult for us to determine the *rate* of change. **Smoothing** is a process that removes the higher frequency (spikes) and allows more of the underlying direction to show through.

Figure 7.1 shows a data graph that has a relatively high level of variability. The first question we would be asked is, "Are we getting better or worse?" We can eyeball the graph and probably respond that the number of late medications appears to be increasing. Our eyeball assessment is not really satisfying; we would rather be able to give a more concrete response.

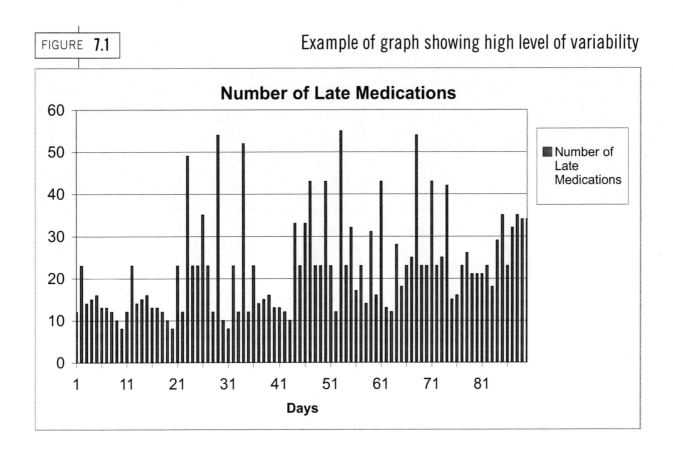

FIGURE **7.1**   Example of graph showing high level of variability

The first easy step in getting that concrete response is to add a smoothed trend line to the graph that eliminates some of the spikes and looks for the underlying trend. Rolling or moving averages are a good tool to use for this.

With rolling or moving averages, instead of plotting a single point on the graph, you average a series of points and you use that average value as a point. If you use a backward-looking, 30-day moving average, the data point for Day 30 would be the average of all the values from Day 1 through Day 29. Then the data point for Day 31 would be an average of all the values from Day 2 through Day 30, and so on.

Figure 7.2 shows a moving average trend line overlaid on the data. Note that the trend line only starts at Period 30. That's normal. It takes the first 30 periods to "prime the pump," so there really can't be a backward-looking moving average before Day 30.

The larger the number of periods that are included in the moving average, the less variability there will be in the line. Try different numbers of periods to get a better understanding of the trend in the direction of the data. The sidebar in this chapter provides an easy way to calculate moving averages in Excel.

FIGURE 7.2 The same chart showing a moving average trend line

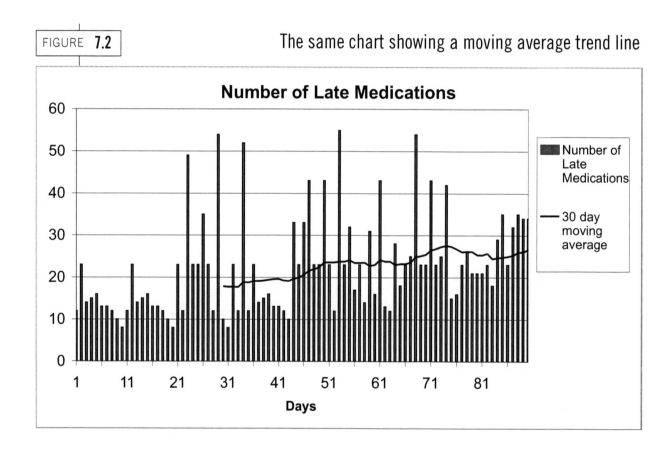

Using crossing averages

In Figure 7.2, the 30-day moving average trend line gives us greater confidence that the number of late medications has increased over the past two months.

If we don't have a clear external benchmark to compare this performance against, we can use an internal benchmark and compare our present performance to our past performance. We do that by using a technique that is often used in the stock market and in investment analysis. This tool is called a "crossing average." The concept of the crossing average is simple but powerful—we compare a short-term moving average with a long-term moving average, see which is on top, and watch for times when these averages "cross."

If our short-term moving average is doing better than our long-term moving average, we are improving. If the opposite is true (i.e., the long-term average is better than the short-term average), our performance is declining. The point at which those two averages cross is a critical time. Either we have lost momentum and are now in a period of declining performance or, if the averages cross in the other direction, we are entering a period of improvement. This gives us a good method to help answer that critical question, "Are we getting better?"

In Figure 7.3, notice that during the past two months the data consistently indicates that the short-term average has been worse than the long-term average. There appears to have been a general decline in delivering medications on time during this period.

FIGURE **7.3**

Crossing averages

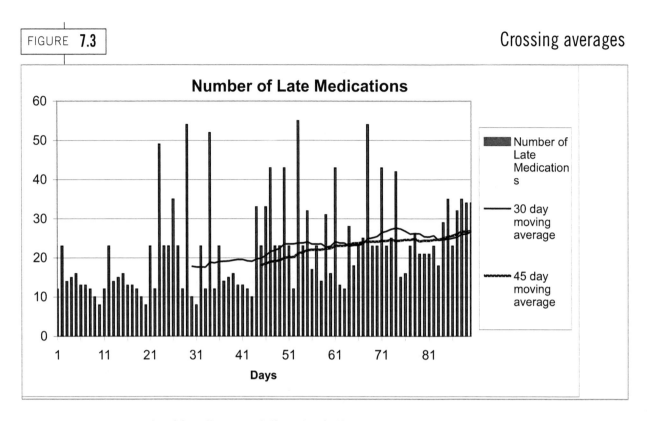

Annotating trends with callouts and direction indicators

Your trend graph is starting to take shape. Now you just need to make it easy to understand and make sure that it communicates your conclusions. To make trend graphs communicate well, you need to *annotate* them with at least the following:

- **A clear indication of which direction is the "good" direction:** If you don't make it clear which direction is the "good" direction, people will be confused when they try to convert the direction of the trend into good or bad. Put an arrow, a label, or a marker on all your graphs to make sure that people can tell which direction is good.

- **Clear indicators of "acceptable" vs. "unacceptable":** Just like you put control limits on control charts, consider putting an indicator of "Acceptable" or "Unacceptable" bands on your graphs.

- **Callouts to make sure that the conclusions are communicated:** Don't force the users of your graph to draw their own conclusions when you have already reached a conclusion. Tell end-users what the data means to them. Too often, the folks who prepare the data graphs think that it will be immediately and intuitively obvious to readers what the graphs mean. Don't assume that—help users by helping the data speak loudly and clearly (see Figure 7.4).

FIGURE **7.4** Example of an annotated graph

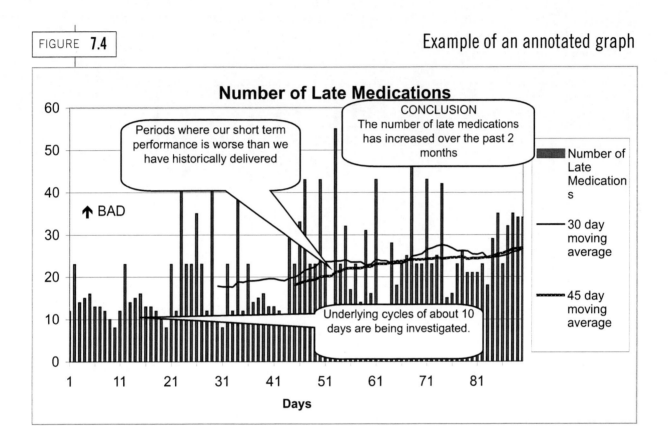

What if you can't draw a conclusion? That's a good test. If you are familiar with the data and you can't draw a conclusion, there is little hope that others will be able to. Maybe that data doesn't have anything to communicate. If that is the case, be careful to not waste people's time with graphs that are not communicating messages that can be used to validate or improve your performance.

 If you can't draw a conclusion from your data, it is unlikely that others will be able to do so, either.

Sidebar: Creating quick-and-dirty moving averages in Excel

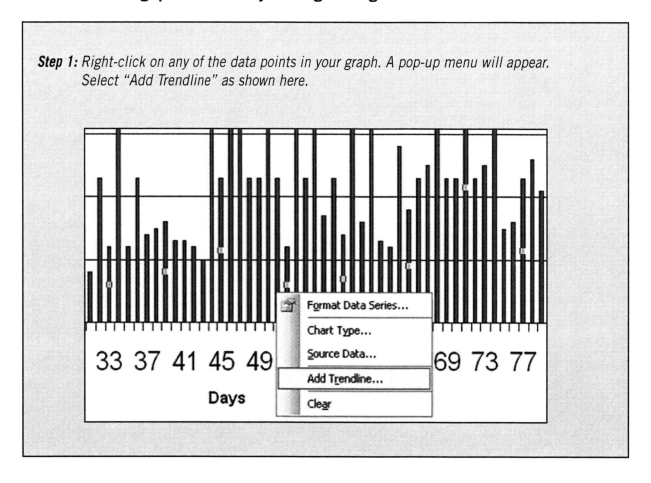

Step 1: *Right-click on any of the data points in your graph. A pop-up menu will appear. Select "Add Trendline" as shown here.*

Creating quick-and-dirty moving averages in Excel (cont.)

Step 2: *Select "Moving Average," and enter the number of periods you would like to average. Make sure that your data is evenly distributed. The Excel Moving Average function just looks at the past 30 periods and will not know whether days are missing. If your data is not evenly (periodically) distributed, you will have to calculate the moving average and plot it, rather than using the graph function.*

Warning: Be careful using Excel moving averages. Make sure that your data is complete and evenly distributed (with no missing days or months). Remember, you are limited to 255 periods.

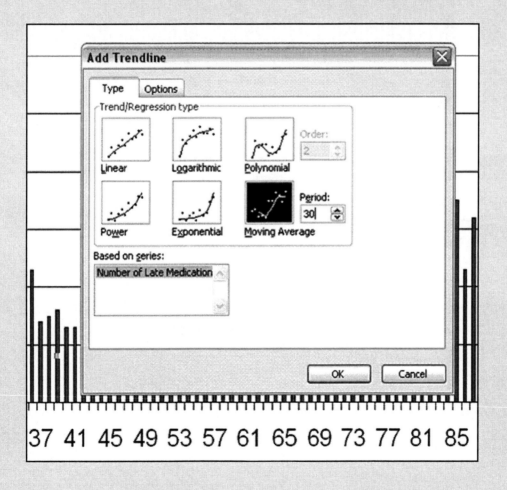

Creating quick-and-dirty moving averages in Excel (cont.)

Step 3: *Format your trend line so that it is useful. To change the line color or its thickness, right-click on the trend line and select "Format Trendline."*

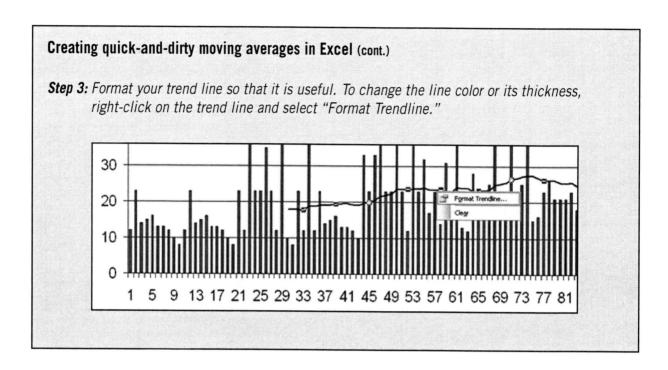

Example: Are your management trends lying to you?

To be effective in causing appropriate change within the organization, management needs to trust the messages that your trend data is whispering or shouting to them. Unfortunately, if you are not careful, your trend process can lead the organization astray.

Figure 7.5 shows a typical data chart that might be presented in a committee meeting or to the board of directors. It is a time-series trend showing how this parameter has changed over time. Unfortunately, it is hard to tell whether this chart is indicating good or bad news. There are no comparison lines, and you have to figure out the trend in your mind.

 Making Your Data Work

FIGURE **7.5**   Typical data chart

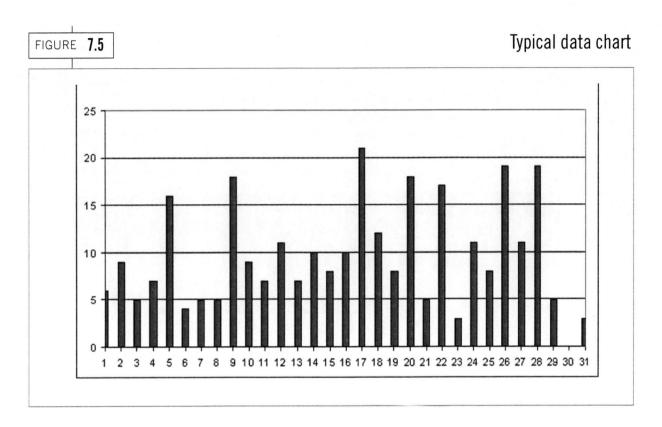

Your next step would be to add bands that clearly indicate whether the data is acceptable or unacceptable, as in Figure 7.6. Doing so also helps others to understand whether "up" is good or bad. It starts to make the story a little clearer, but the graph still is not talking to you.

Data chart with bands

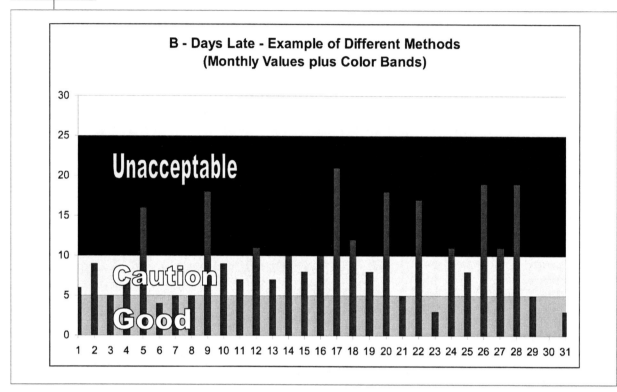

Now, you might be tempted to convert the graph into a dashboard to help communicate more clearly. This is basically a good idea, but you need to make sure that it helps you understand the message. Figure 7.7 is an example of a dashboard or annunciator chart that you might create. It shows which band you are in (shown here as dark gray, gray, or light gray, but you would probably use colors) and in which direction you are moving.

On first blush, this seems like it would be useful. But look at the signal that is being sent to the control loop: "getting worse," "getting better," "getting worse," "getting better." Those arrows are changing direction almost every month.

FIGURE **7.7**   Example of a dashboard or annunciator chart

	Monthly	Numerical trend direction
6		↓
7		↓
8		--
9		↓
10		↑
11		↑
12		↓
13		↑
14		↓
15		↑
16		↓
17		↓
18		↑
19		↑
20		↓
21		↑
22		↓
23		↑
24		↓
25		↑
26		↓
27		↑
28		↓
29		↑
30		↑
31		↓

Caution: If you send this kind of signal to your management (control loop), you are setting them up to oscillate back and forth without really knowing whether they are doing the right thing. That often leads to knee-jerk responses and "Program-of-the-Month" solutions. If this were a machine, such a series of signals being sent to the control loop might wear out the machine or, even worse, cause it to break down.

Using this data, could you confidently answer the key question, "Should we stay the course or change direction?" If you can't, it is unlikely that the data will be useful to your leadership team or to the department managers. You need to do something to smooth out all those oscillations.

Therefore, your next step is to use a moving average to help you filter out the variability and see the underlying trend. Using a short-term (six-month) moving average, you can clearly see that the trend is worsening and get some idea of the rate. It also is clear that your facility is in the "unacceptable" band and has been there for a while (see Figure 7.8).

FIGURE **7.8**   Example of a moving average that shows worsening performance

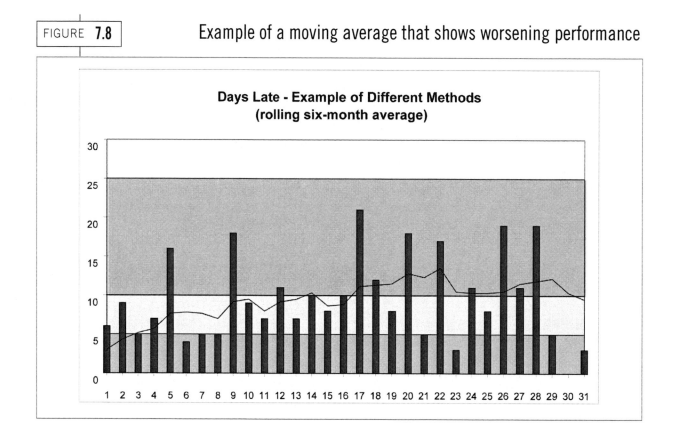

Now let's add a second moving average—this time, a 12-month average (see Figure 7.9). Now you can use the crossing average tool and compare the short- and long-term moving averages.

FIGURE **7.9** Example of data chart with two moving averages

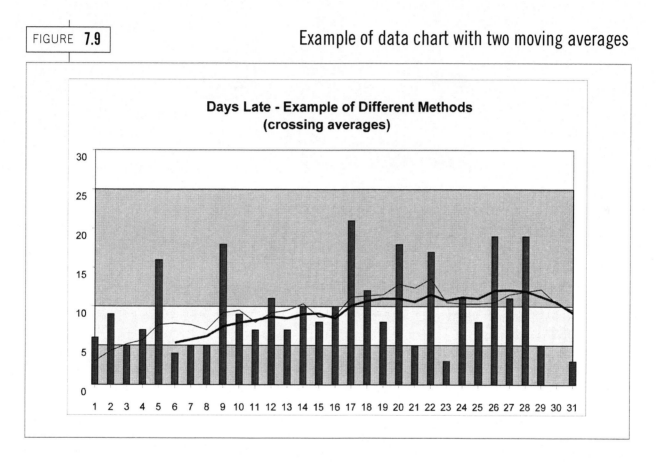

Now you have three pieces of information that you can use to help communicate with your departments, senior leaders, or the board. You know whether the present value is in the acceptable or unacceptable band, and you know the short-term moving average and the long-term moving average.

Figure 7.10 uses the same dashboard layout (monthly color with direction indicator), but this time the moving averages have been used to select the color and the direction.

FIGURE **7.10**   Same data, different analysis, questions answered

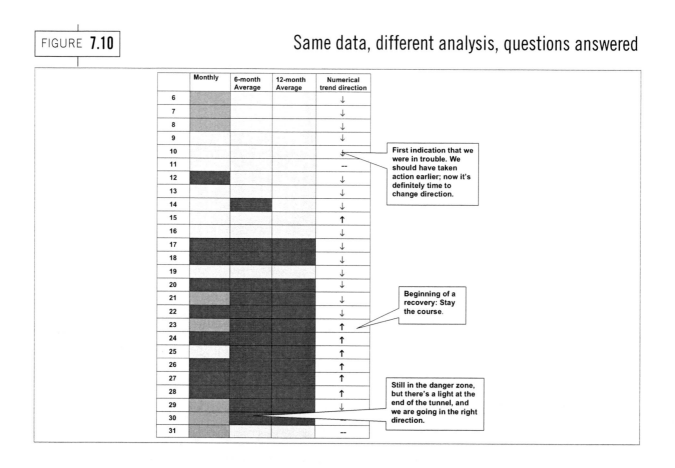

Immediately, we see that we were in the "caution" band for 10 months, from months 6 through 16, and we were consistently declining in performance. How do we know we were declining in performance? We know that because the short-term moving average was above (worse than) the long-term moving average. This indicates that we are not doing as well as we have historically demonstrated we could.

Now think about the control signal you are sending to leadership: "We have been in a caution state for 10 months, and every month we are getting worse. Is there any surprise that we ended up in the danger zone?"

Wouldn't it be easier to answer that key question now? "We need to change direction because if we keep doing this, we will not improve."

At month 17, your organization slides into the danger zone, and performance continues to decline.

Now maybe you have the organization's attention and they start to respond. By month 23, you see that finally you have turned the corner and are starting to do better than you have been doing in the past. You have a series of six months of continuous improvement (although you're still in the danger zone). Then you have a bad result in month 29. How would you answer your key question? You probably have enough data to be able to say, "Stay the course. It was a bad month, but we are going in the right direction."

Figure 7.11 compares these two techniques. The same data can send either a confusing signal or a useful signal. It's up to you!

FIGURE **7.11**   Same data, different analysis

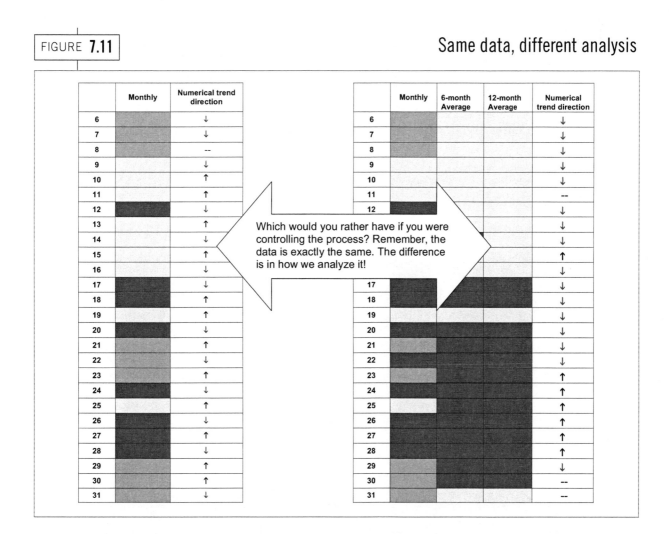

Use your moving averages, direction indicators, and annotations to send clear messages to your leadership.

Make trending work: Hold regular trend meetings

In process and information management, there is the concept of "push" and "pull." *Push* means that we decide what someone needs or wants, and we push that data out to him or her. *Pull* means that the user decides what is useful to him or her, and the user gets the opportunity to "pull" the data he or she needs at that moment. E-mailing a trend report to the CNO is a push, whereas someone searching for a specific topic he or she is interested in is a pull.

One failure that often occurs in a trend program is that we rely too heavily on pushing data—we decide what to trend, we make the graphs, and we tell the end-user what he or she should do about it. Not only does this "insulate" the end-user from the data, but it also often results in pushback: "You don't know my department! How can you be telling me what my problems are?"

A program that relies on pushing data can also be frustrating to the data management folks. We analyze the data, make nice charts and graphs, send out many pages of data, and sometimes are not even sure whether anyone looks at the material, let alone uses it to make changes.

Whenever possible in your trend program, set up the process so that the end users have control over the flow of information and can develop their own "aha's!" One effective way to do this is to schedule regular trend review meetings and interactively share the data, rather than relying on printed graphs.

How can you do that? Figure 7.12 provides an example of how to improve the number of new insights that you glean from your occurrence report data through an interactive trend meeting.

FIGURE **7.12**   Make your trend meetings more effective

**Example of how to use bi-monthly trend review meetings to improve your
occurrence report analysis**

❑ Export your occurrence data from your data-tracking system (MIDAS, STARs, QUANTROS, etc.) to Excel.

❑ Add columns to help you analyze and trend the data:

   - Convert the Date field to Month, Year, and Day

   - Convert the Severity field to a numerical value (weighted significance)

❑ Build a pivot table/pivot chart (see Chapter 8).

❑ Set up a meeting with the key department (Nursing, Pharmacy, Lab, Registration, etc.).

❑ Use the drag-and-drop capabilities of the pivot tables to show the high-level trends to the group. Get them engaged!

❑ Show the data as histograms and then as a time series. Then zoom in on key contributors.

❑ Watch as the departments start to ask questions. For example, "Can you show me that by shift?" "Which floor has the largest number of . . . ?"

❑ Record the "aha's" that the departments come up with, and ask them what they think should happen next (trigger the action).

❑ Follow up in two months with the next trend meeting, revisit the "aha's" from last time, and look for more.

Assist the departments in discovering their own "aha's" by having regularly scheduled trend review meetings.

Endnotes

1. For more information about the FMEA process, see Rohde, K.R., *Failure Modes and Effect Analysis: Templates and Tools to Improve Patient Safety* Marblehead, MA: HCPro, Inc., 2007.

Common Cause Analysis and the Significant Event Database

Managing your significant event data via common cause analysis

In Chapter 1, we established that effective management of exception (problem) data was a key aspect of an effective control loop. In this chapter, we will look at how we manage a very important subset of the exception data: your *significant event data.*

A typical medium-size hospital may collect 3,000 to 8,000 exception or occurrence reports every year. These are usually self-reported and cover a large variety of different areas, including medication errors, falls, treatment problems, security issues, and often many others.

We know that all of these occurrences did not have the same impact on the patients or the organization. Some were minor, some were early warnings, and others were very serious or "significant." Some of the exceptions we will just "trend," but others, especially the more significant ones, will require more attention (see Figure 8.1).

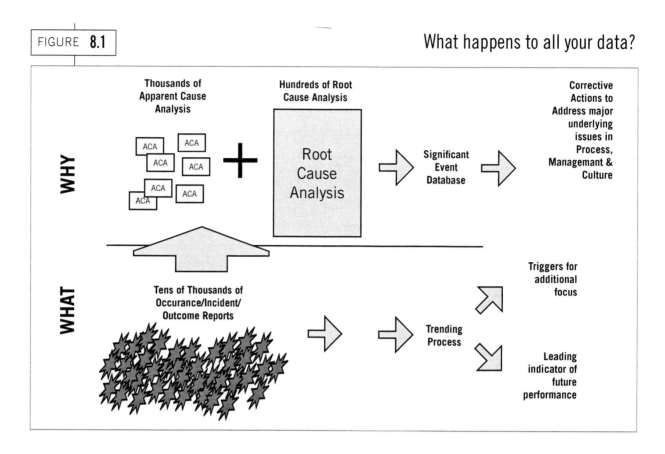

FIGURE 8.1 What happens to all your data?

So what makes an event significant? Generally, an event is considered significant if the consequences are unacceptable and you want that event (and its cousins) to never happen again. The Joint Commission classifies a group of these events as sentinel events, or events that are warnings of serious potential trouble in the organization. You should view these externally defined sentinel events as well as the "Never Events" defined by the National Quality Forum as a subset of the bigger set of events that are "significant" to your organization.

Management of "significant event" data requires that, at a minimum, we be able to do two things well:

- Perform a meta-analysis of all significant events to look for underlying common causes

- Graphically demonstrate a reduction in the impact of significant events over time

In this chapter, we will focus on these two key aspects of managing our data.

   Making Your Data Work

What is common cause analysis?

Whenever we have an event that results in consequences that we want to prevent from happening again, we conduct a causal analysis, sometimes called a root cause analysis (RCA), to determine why the specific event happened. These analyses have now generated "why" data that we need to manage.

This "why" data is some of the most "refined" and valuable data that we will have, but often it is "unmanaged," and as a result, we are not able to rely on our data in a critical area.

Think about your organization. Can you assist your organization by helping it to see the underlying differences, commonalities, and similarities between the past 20 cause analyses that the organization has performed? If you can, you are providing real, meaningful information that will assist in changing the way you do business.

If we focus only on individual events, we are just picking dandelion tops. Wait a few days and there will be more (both dandelions and problems!). But if we can dig down and find bigger, more common issues that are "generating" our problems, and if we can fix those issues, we will be making real progress.

 Consider your significant event data as some of the most useful and valuable information you will handle.

Figure 8.2 shows the daily problems at the top—some of which are significant enough that we investigate them more fully using a cause analysis method—often RCA or apparent cause analysis (ACA). Common Cause Analysis is just a specialized analysis of our histogram or binned data to help us see commonalities in the results of our cause analyses.

FIGURE **8.2**

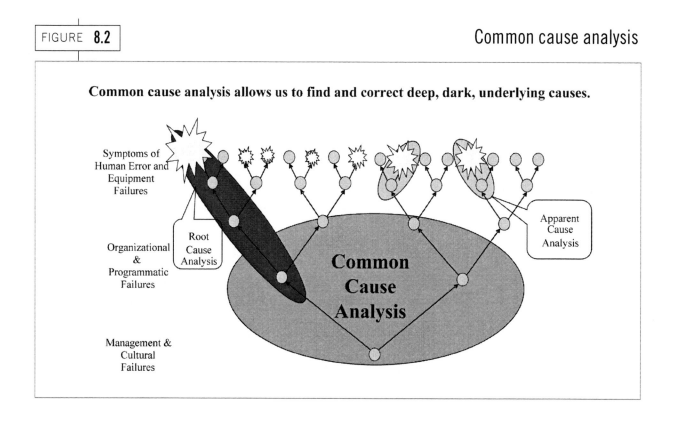

Common cause analysis allows us to find and correct deep, dark, underlying causes.

Symptoms of Human Error and Equipment Failures

Root Cause Analysis

Organizational & Programmatic Failures

Common Cause Analysis

Apparent Cause Analysis

Management & Cultural Failures

The significant event database (SEDB)

The first step in getting your significant event data under control is to get it all in one place. This means that the quality, risk, and data analysis functions need to work together and collect the results of all the cause analyses in one place in a standard format. Sounds easy, and technically, it is easy, but many organizations haven't been able to get over this first hurdle. Internal turf battles and concerns about discovery and protection sometimes result in significant event data being held very tightly and not shared or analyzed in aggregate. This is very unfortunate, because it often results in slowing our progress in preventing the recurrence of the events we most want to keep from ever happening again.

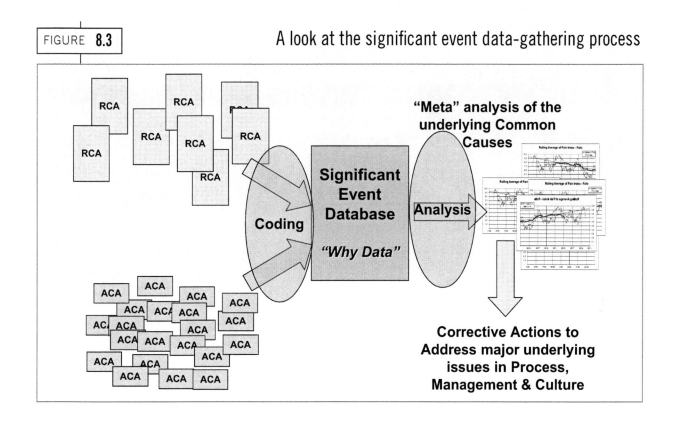

FIGURE **8.3**   A look at the significant event data-gathering process

Set up a formal process to collect the key information from each significant event and store it in the SEDB.

The SEDB can be as simple as an Excel spreadsheet or as complicated as your resources allow. A simple spreadsheet is really all you need (see Figure 8.4), so don't go overboard on the database. The goal is to collect, code, and analyze the causal factors that are uncovered in your cause analysis.

FIGURE **8.4**   Typical fields in the SEDB

Typical field	Contents
Cause analysis number	This is a code that connects the data back to your RCA, ACA, or occurrence report.
Causal factor number	Just a sequence number (1, 2, 3, etc.); there may be 8-10 causal factors that were uncovered in each of the cause analyses.
Title of event	So that you can remember what the event was.
Brief description of event	Fifty to 100 words to describe the event. If you are looking at the data two years after the event occurred, this will help you to understand the causal factors.
Causal factor	A brief description of the "why" that contributed to or caused the event. There may be 8-10 of these.
Department/location	The department or location where the action that resulted in the causal factor occurred.
Process	The process being used that was connected with the causal factor.
Activity	The activity being performed that was connected with the causal factor.
Error type	A human error, process error, or equipment error.
Error code(s)	Multiple fields that code and roll up the error description.
Expectation not met	Tie it back to your Culture of Safety Expectations for Safe Behaviors, Good Equipment, and Process Management.
Corrective action description	A description of what was to be done about the causal factor.
Corrective action type	Use this to sort your corrective actions (procedure change, training, peer review, improved equipment, etc.)
Corrective action strength	Are the corrective actions proposed "transitory" or "permanent"?
Process being corrected	Use this to demonstrate all the improvements by process at the end of the year. Also, this connects the significant event database to the process management process.

After you have developed and coded your SEDB, use your pivot table and pivot chart tools in Excel (discussed in greater detail in Chapter 9) to start to slice and dice the data in different dimensions, looking for commonalities. Then use those common causes to help the organization identify additional analyses that may be needed to develop effective improvement activities (see Figure 8.5).

FIGURE **8.5**   The common cause analysis process

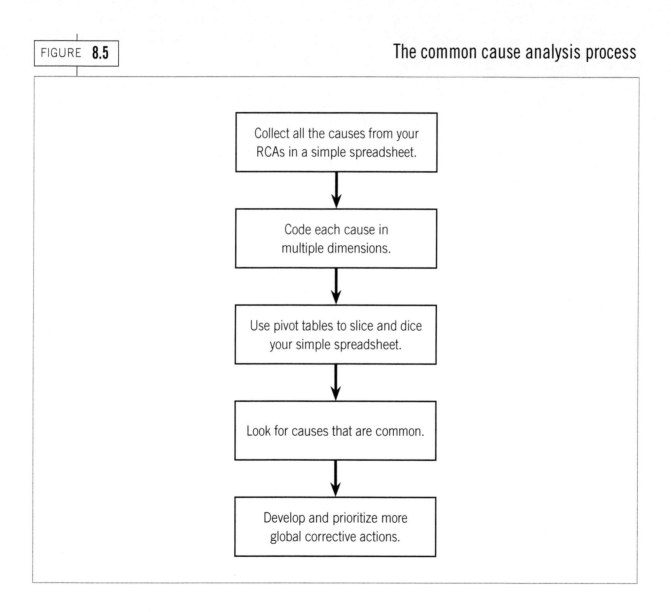

Multidimensional analysis

Multidimensional analysis is just doing a "slice and dice" using multiple pieces of information. For example, if we made three slices through our data—one for the event type, one for the location, and one for bed side rails—we might get an output chart that shows that the largest number of events is "Falls" on "Floor 4 North" with "Bed Side Rails Up." That would be a multidimensional analysis. The more dimensions we can cut our data into, the more useful it is to us. Remember the discussion of codes in Chapter 4? The more effective your codes are, the easier it will be to do multidimensional slices.

Multidimensional slices are a key part of the analysis process; we look for differences and commonalities in these slices. If we identify a difference, that says something has jumped out at us, such as an excessive number of falls on 4 North with the bed side rails up.

If we identify commonalities, we might see that handoffs seem to be causing problems on all the nursing floors. That is telling us that handoffs are a common problem across multiple locations. If we can fix common problems, we get a bigger, faster result because more people will benefit from the solution.

Figure 8.6 shows how you can use charts to perform multidimensional analyses.

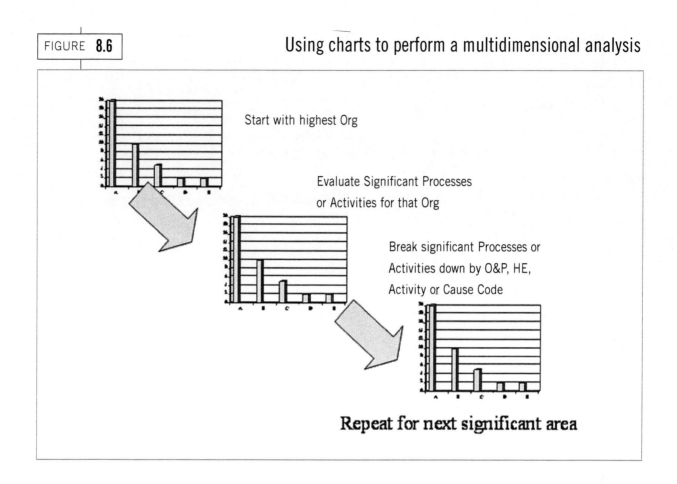

FIGURE **8.6**   Using charts to perform a multidimensional analysis

Start with highest Org

Evaluate Significant Processes
or Activities for that Org

Break significant Processes or
Activities down by O&P, HE,
Activity or Cause Code

Repeat for next significant area

Separating out the "bug dust"

We have sliced and diced the data and have presented the number of occurrences in a histogram chart. Now, how can we start to draw conclusions from this data?

We need a series of methods that will help us to determine whether something is important and may indicate a difference in our data set. We need to make sure that we are not looking at "bug dust," those small but annoying pieces of information that don't really help us.

There are many ways to determine whether data is statistically significant, but here we are just going to look at ways to screen data to determine whether there are commonalities and differences.

Use some formal cutoff line to keep out of the "bug dust."

The following would indicate differences in your histogram chart:

- A natural break between the large contributors and small contributors that is apparent through direct examination

- The 80% contribution as indicated on the Pareto chart cumulative line

- Any contributors with a confidence indicator greater than 80%, and especially if the confidence indicator is greater than 99%

Figure 8.7 describes these three methods. Figure 8.8 shows how to determine what data is important and what is merely bug dust in a histogram.

FIGURE **8.7**   Separating the vital few from the rest

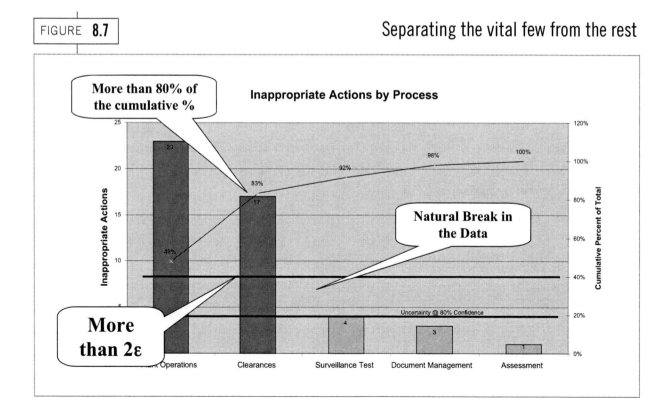

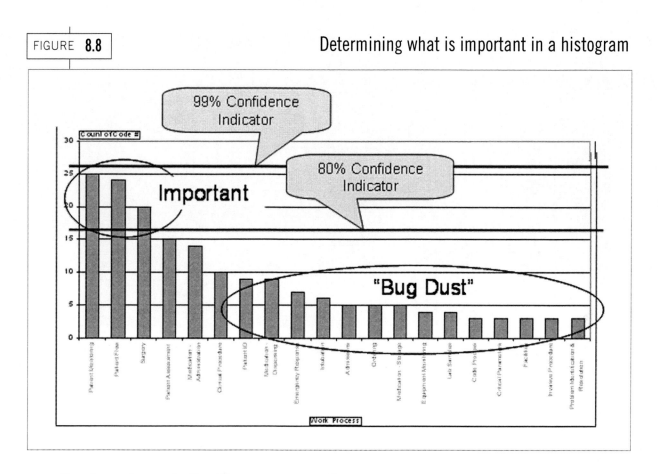

FIGURE 8.8   Determining what is important in a histogram

How do you know whether things are common?

When you plot your histogram, make multidimensional slices through it, and see a "plateau" where multiple values are all about the same, that is an indication that there may be an underlying commonality.

Figures 8.9 and 8.10 show what histograms might look like for isolated problems and for common problems.

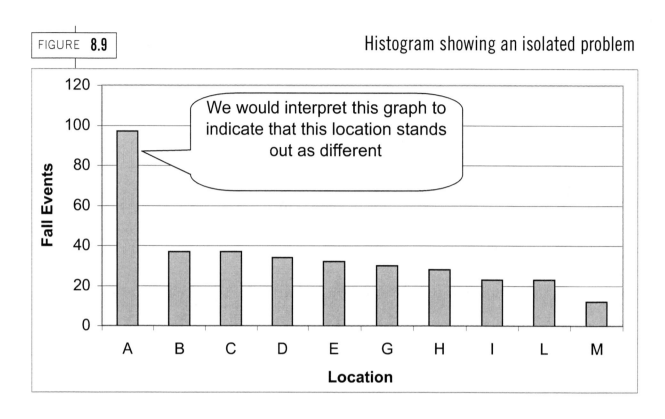

FIGURE **8.9**

Histogram showing an isolated problem

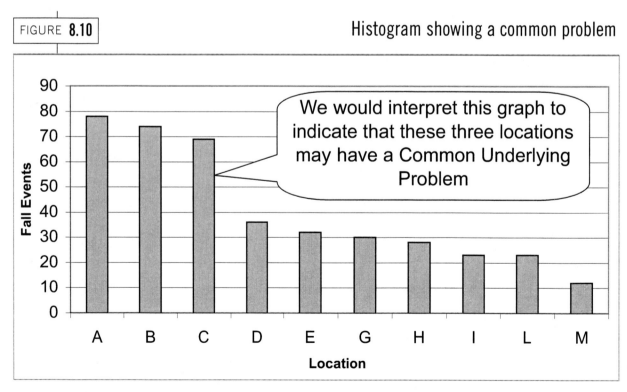

FIGURE **8.10**

Histogram showing a common problem

Making Your Data Work

The goal with the common cause analysis is to look through all of our multidimensional slices and find areas that are more likely to be common underlying problems. If we fix the common underlying problems, we will have a greater benefit.

Graphically demonstrating a reduction in the impact of your significant events

One of the key areas we are usually asked to analyze is our rate of improvement, especially in the reduction of our significant events. You can use several methods to demonstrate your improvement, as shown in Figure 8.11. Choose one or two that best communicate within your organization.

FIGURE **8.11**   Problem-solving methods and considerations

Methods to Demonstrate Reductions in Significant Events	
Method	**Things to consider**
Significant event rate reduction: *Number of significant events per x patient days*	This method is often used, and it normalizes based on volume, but it sends the hidden message that "the busier we are, the more acceptable significant events are." This may not be a healthy message.
Rate of reduction of significant events: *The percentage of fewer significant events compared to last year*	This doesn't need to be normalized because it is a ratio. It is a good continuous indicator.
Absolute number of significant events: *We had 30 last year, and we have had 12 this year. We are getting better.*	This is a good method. Don't worry too much about the lack of normalization. Be proud if you can reduce the absolute number of people who are being harmed.
Ratio of significant events to all events: *Five percent of our reported events used to be significant events. Now only 3.5% are significant events.*	This isolates people from the real harm and is very dependent on changes in the reporting rate. Consider combining this with average severity per report instead.
Time between significant events: *We have gone 156 days since our last significant event.*	This can be demoralizing every time the clock resets.
Average severity per report.	Although this includes more than just significant events, it is a very useful, high-level method to indicate improvement or decline.

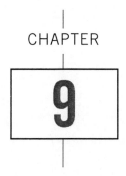
Pivot Tables: The Data Analyst's Best Friend

Understanding data structures

To help your organization get the most value out of the data it collects, you need to be able to rapidly and efficiently manipulate your data so that it reveals its real value.

Unfortunately, we often become overwhelmed by our data and by the effort it seems to require to do even the simplest analysis or make "just one more table" for management or a department.

Data analysis is resource-intensive, but some tools can help us significantly to deliver results more quickly. Pivot tables and pivot charts hold real value for your data analysis team because they can convert a linear list into a two-dimensional table using simple drag-and-drop functions.

The pivot table and pivot chart creation features found in Excel (Under the "Data" menu, select Pivot Table, Pivot Chart Report) are good examples of such resources. Even many experienced data analysis veterans might not be familiar with these powerful tools.

Linear data sets vs. two-dimensional data tables

When we think of a data table, we think of a two-dimensional array, perhaps with the names of departments going down one side and the months going across the top. Managers and committees often like to see data presented in this way, so you manually add all the data and type it into the row and column in your spreadsheet, and you e-mail it off. Done!

But then they ask a question: "Could I see this by floor?" Your stomach tightens because you know you have to do the whole process over again. Either you work overtime or you try to talk them out of data that might result in an "Aha" revelation.

Isn't there a better way?

There certainly is, but it depends on us changing our approach to managing data. We need to stop managing data in a two-dimensional table and instead think about a two-step process in which:

1. We manage our data in a linear list.

2. We automatically generate two-dimensional tables from that linear list.

The tool that allows us to automatically generate these two-dimensional tables is the Excel function for pivot tables and pivot charts.

How do we do this?

Let's look at a chart of falls data. In Figure 9.1, we have the weighted significance of falls by month and location.

We might be tempted to manage our data in this two-dimensional table with months across the top and locations down the left side. The problem with this approach is that there is no place to go next. We have painted ourselves into a corner, and any question will require us to start from scratch. The real underlying problem is that we have more than one value of related information on the same row in our spreadsheet. We have multiple values for the Month field—that is, data for both March and April in the same row.

FIGURE **9.1**

A two-dimensional table limits your flexibility

Weighted Severity of Falls	2006						2006 Total
Location	Jul	Aug	Sep	Oct	Nov	Dec	
5 North					95		95
ED	25	70	70				165
FRONT LOBBY					35	25	60
HALLWAY							
HOME/RESIDENCE		35	70				105
PATIENT ROOM		35	70		160	70	335
RADIOGRAPHICS			35	35		35	105
REHAB SERVICES	60			60			120
Total Falls	85	140	245	95	290	130	985

A simple linear list would have a separate row for each piece of related information. In Figure 9.2, notice that there is a new row every time the data changes.

FIGURE **9.2**
Managing your data in a linear list

Incident Year	Incident Month	Location	Outcome	Weighted Significance
2006	7	ED	ABRASION	25
2006	7	REHAB SERVICES	Unknown	35
2006	7	REHAB SERVICES	NO APPARENT INJURY	25
2006	8	ED	Unknown	35
2006	8	ED	CONTUSION	35
2006	8	HOME/RESIDENCE	LACERATION	35
2006	8	PATIENT ROOM	NO APPARENT INJURY	35
2006	9	ED	CONTUSION	35
2006	9	ED	LACERATION	35
2006	9	HOME/RESIDENCE	LACERATION	35
2006	9	HOME/RESIDENCE	SKIN TEARS	35
2006	9	PATIENT ROOM	Unknown	35
2006	9	PATIENT ROOM	NO APPARENT INJURY	35
2006	9	RADIOGRAPHICS	UNKNOWN OUTCOME	35
2006	10	RADIOGRAPHICS	FRACTURE	35
2006	10	REHAB SERVICES	Unknown	25
2006	10	REHAB SERVICES	PAIN	35
2006	11	5 North	NO APPARENT INJURY	60
2006	11	6 North	REDNESS	35
2006	11	FRONT LOBBY	CONTUSION	35
2006	11	PATIENT ROOM	ABRASION	35
2006	11	PATIENT ROOM	CONTUSION	35
2006	11	PATIENT ROOM	NO APPARENT INJURY	40
2006	11	PATIENT ROOM	PAIN	25
2006	11	PATIENT ROOM	SCRATCH	25
2006	12	FRONT LOBBY	NO APPARENT INJURY	25
2006	12	PATIENT ROOM	NO APPARENT INJURY	70
2006	12	RADIOGRAPHICS	NO APPARENT INJURY	35
2007	1	ED	ABRASION	25

 Making Your Data Work

Now the data in Figure 9.2 may not be in the form you want to present, but that's easy to fix. Next, you would simply convert the linear list to a two-dimensional table using the pivot table function in Excel. You get the output table your managers want, and if they ask a question such as "Can I see that by outcome?" all you have to do is drag the Outcome field onto the pivot table, and you are done. (See Figure 9.3.) This takes little of your time, your audience thinks you are a genius, and hopefully everyone gets an important "aha" from the process. See the step-by-step instructions at the end of this chapter.

FIGURE **9.3**   Table automatically generated by the Excel Pivot Table function

Sum of Weighted Severity			2006					
Incident Category	Location	Outcome	7	8	9	10	11	12
Fall	5 North	ABRASION						
		NO APPARENT INJURY					60	
		REDNESS					35	
	ED	ABRASION	25					
		CONTUSION		35	35			
		LACERATION			35			
		NO APPARENT INJURY						
	FRONT LOBBY	ABRASION						
		CONTUSION					35	
		NO APPARENT INJURY						25
		PAIN						
	HALLWAY	ABRASION						
		NO APPARENT INJURY						
		SCRATCH						
		STRAIN/SPRAIN						
		UNKNOWN OUTCOME						
	HOME/ RESIDENCE	LACERATION		35	35			
		SKIN TEARS			35			
	PATIENT ROOM	ABRASION					35	
		CONTUSION					35	
		NO APPARENT INJURY		35	35		40	70
		PAIN					25	

Try to keep your data in linear data sets, and then use pivot tables to convert the linear data sets into two-dimensional tables.

The following sidebar describes the steps for creating pivot charts and pivot tables in Excel.

Step by step: How to use pivot tables and pivot charts

Following is a step-by-step process to create a pivot table or pivot chart. The version of Excel that you are using may differ slightly from this, but these steps should be very similar for most Excel users.

Pivot tables and charts are easy to use once you learn the basics—and they really are the data analyst's best friend!

Step 1: *Initial worksheet*

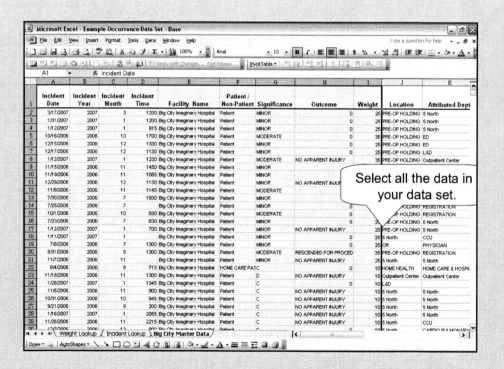

Step 2: *Select Data* ➤ *Pivot Table*

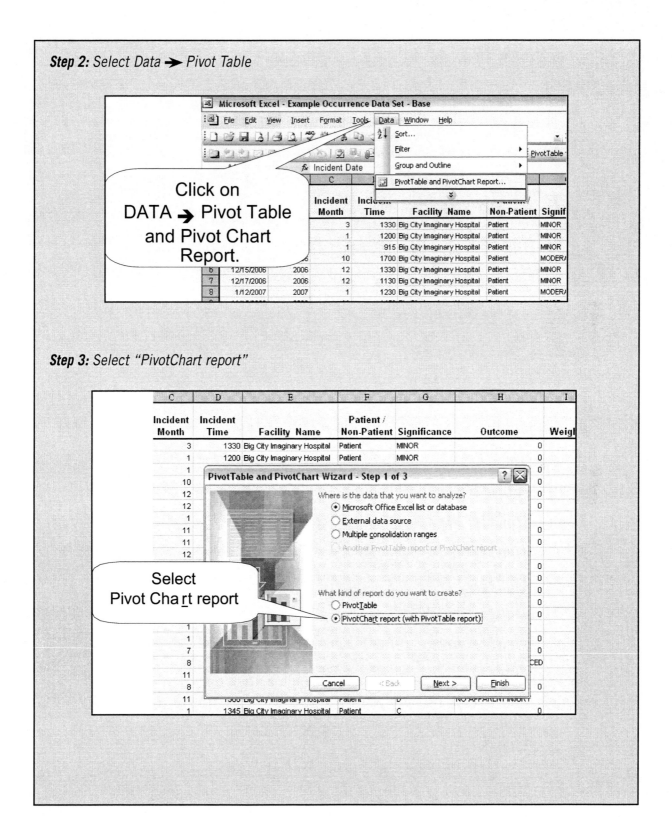

Step 3: *Select "PivotChart report"*

Step 4: *Set the data range, if you have not already done so.*

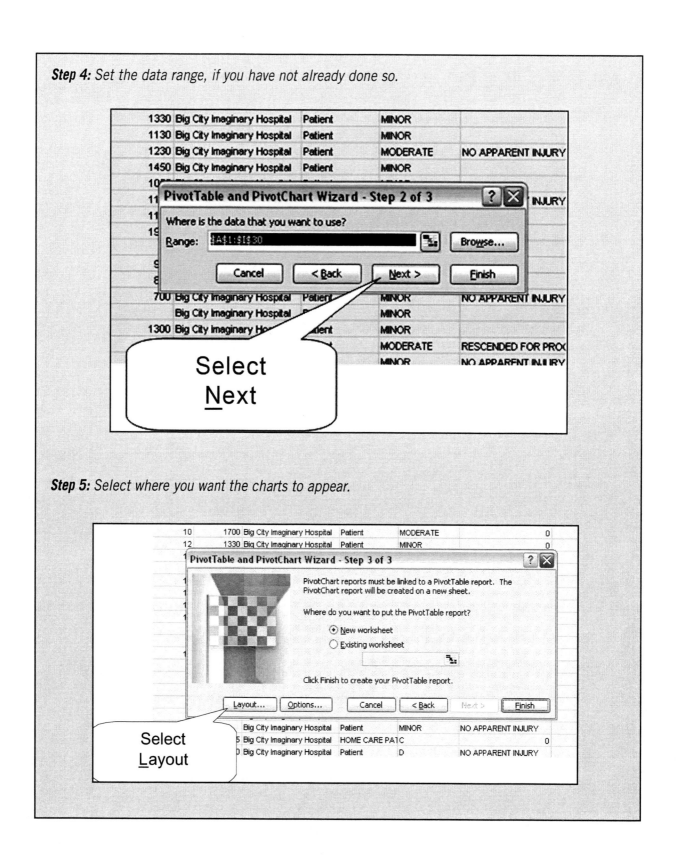

Step 5: *Select where you want the charts to appear.*

Step 6: *Don't worry too much about the initial layout.*

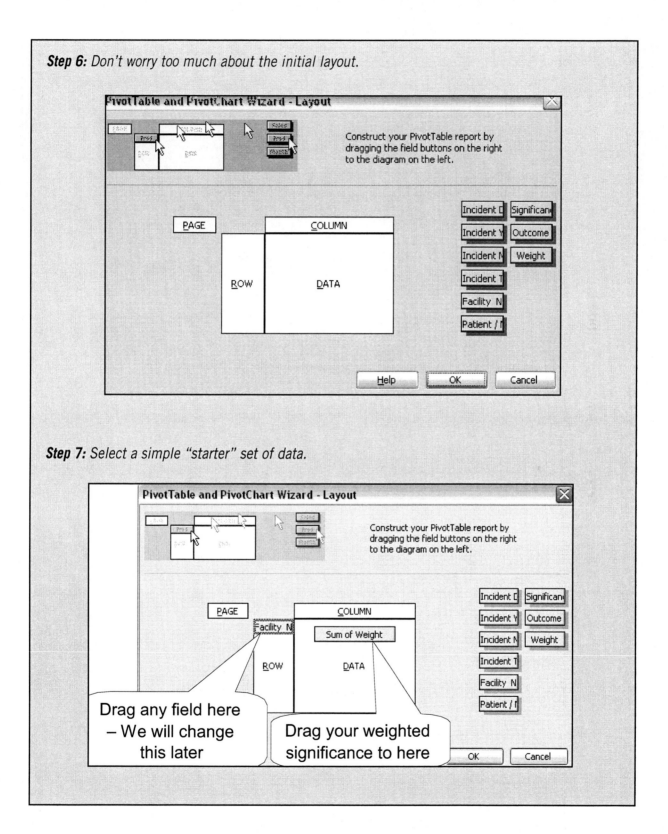

Step 7: *Select a simple "starter" set of data.*

Step 8: *Click Finish to make the pivot table and chart.*

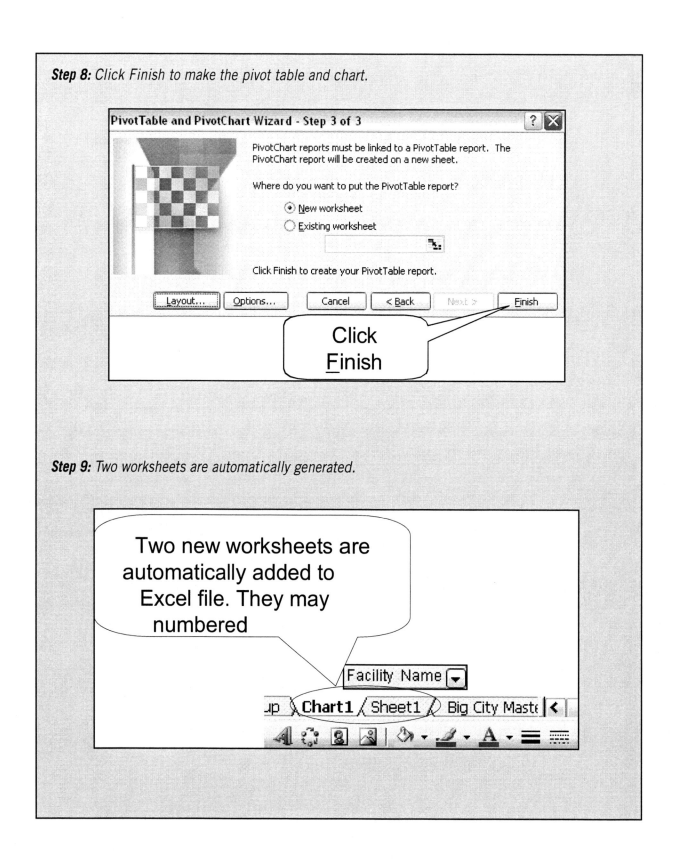

Step 9: *Two worksheets are automatically generated.*

Step 10: The chart and the sheet.

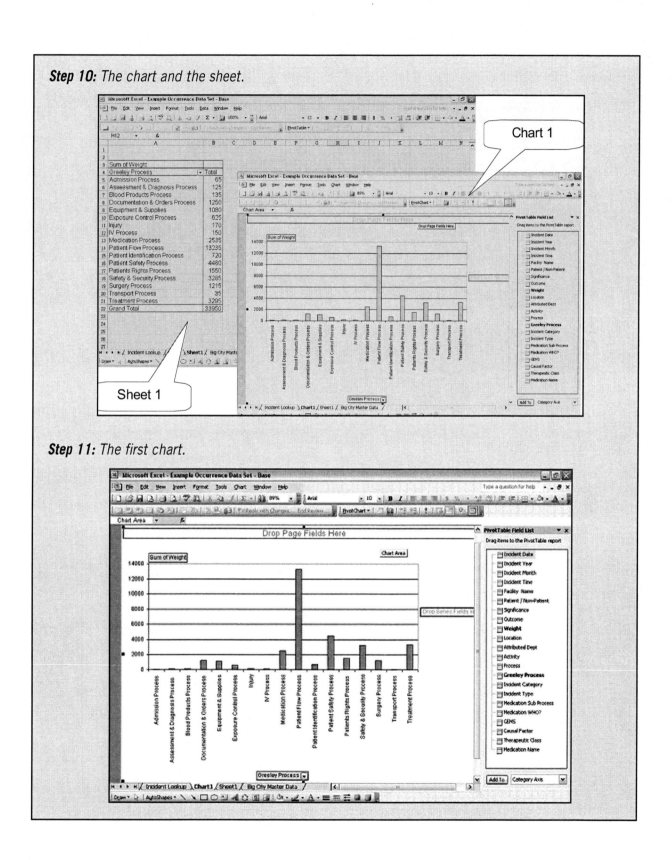

Step 11: The first chart.

Step 12: *Click on the PivotTable option to sort by column and Top 10.*

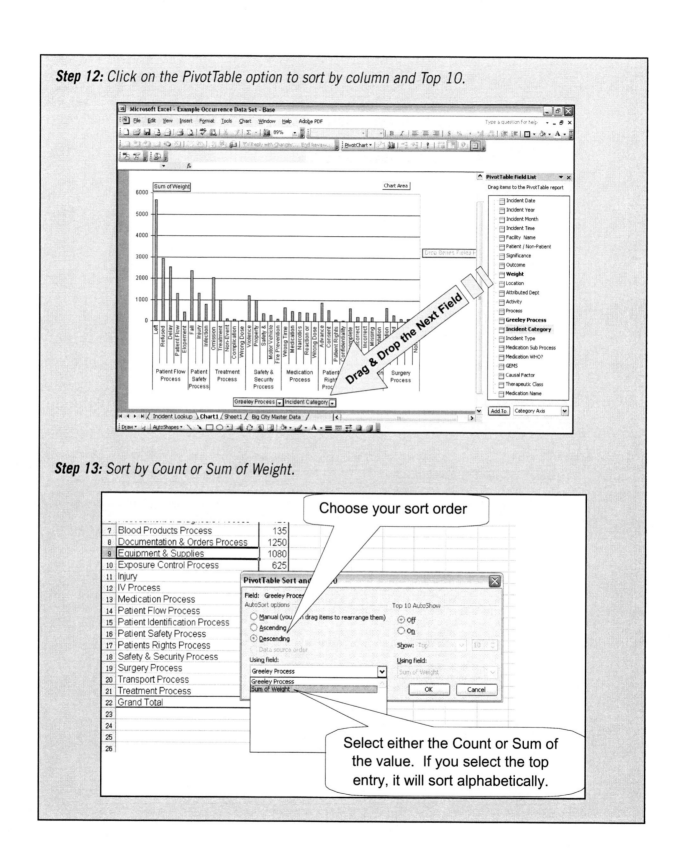

Step 13: *Sort by Count or Sum of Weight.*

CHAPTER

Presenting Your Data

Dashboards, stoplight charts, and displaying your data

If we agree that the real value of a good data program is to collect data, analyze it effectively, and then feed it back to the organization to cause change, the presentation of the data becomes an essential part of the process.

But organizations can fall into traps when they share their data (see Figure 10.1).

 FIGURE **10.1**   Data presentation traps to avoid

> **Trap 1:** Presenting the wrong level of detail to the different levels in the organization
>
> **Trap 2:** Presenting data at the wrong frequency (e.g., quarterly or semiannual data that is "ancient history")
>
> **Trap 3:** Presenting data without conclusions
>
> **Trap 4:** Not indicating what is important and what is "bug dust"
>
> **Trap 5:** Not linking the data with the overall strategy

Choose your presentation methods well to make sure that your data is effective in causing change. Use the checklist in Figure 10.2.

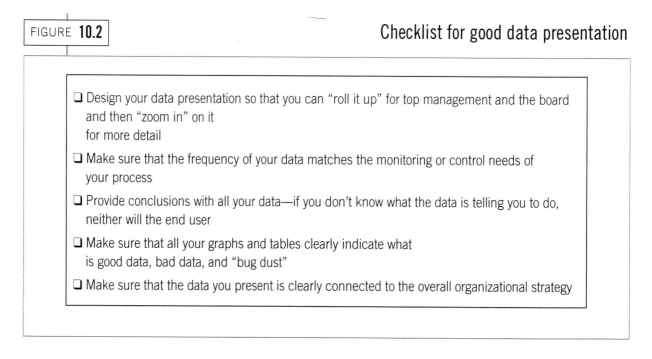

FIGURE **10.2**

Checklist for good data presentation

❑ Design your data presentation so that you can "roll it up" for top management and the board and then "zoom in" on it
for more detail

❑ Make sure that the frequency of your data matches the monitoring or control needs of your process

❑ Provide conclusions with all your data—if you don't know what the data is telling you to do, neither will the end user

❑ Make sure that all your graphs and tables clearly indicate what is good data, bad data, and "bug dust"

❑ Make sure that the data you present is clearly connected to the overall organizational strategy

Using dashboards to present data

We all are familiar with data reports, and we have discussed data graphs in detail in previous chapters. These two workhorses are used all the time. The remaining key method to presenting data effectively—especially for monitoring—is the ***dashboard*** or ***stoplight*** chart.

When you're driving your car, you expect the most important information related to your vehicle to be located within easy view in a clear presentation on the dashboard. In a submarine, airplane, or nuclear power plant control room, all the key information is carefully arranged so that the operators can quickly monitor and control processes.

In healthcare, we need to provide a similarly easy-to-use data display method for our departments, leadership, and boards. Four key things to consider when designing your dashboards are:

- Show absolute "acceptability"

- Show direction and rate of change

- Roll up and roll down

- Match the data detail to the end-user

 Making Your Data Work

Typically in a dashboard, colors are used to display absolute "acceptability." If, for example, an indicator light on the dashboard is red, the corresponding aspect of your car's performance has been judged as "unacceptable."

Dashboards typically use some combination of the following:

- **Blue:** Exceeds expectations

- **Green:** Meets expectations

- **White:** Is within acceptable bounds for external regulators but does not meet internal expectations

- **Yellow:** Falls below acceptable limits

- **Red:** Does not meet minimum requirements

The color, therefore, tells us the status of the indicator or key measure, but it does not help us know at a glance whether we are getting better or worse. Use a directional indicator (such as an up or down arrow) to show the direction of change. Red and getting worse is bad; green and getting better is great!

Next, you need to be able to match the data's level of detail to the end-user. Figure 10.3 provides a top-level dashboard such as one that might be shared with the board of directors. Make sure that each box on the dashboard is really meaningful and is mission-critical to the board.

You can zoom in on each box on the top-level dashboard to see more detail. Figure 10.4 indicates an example of a second-level dashboard. Then you can zoom in on this to the third-level dashboard, and so on. By the time you get below the third level, you probably change over to data graphs and then to data tables as you go into increasing detail.

The third level is also a good place to compare data to benchmarks.

Dashboard styles

FIGURE **10.3**

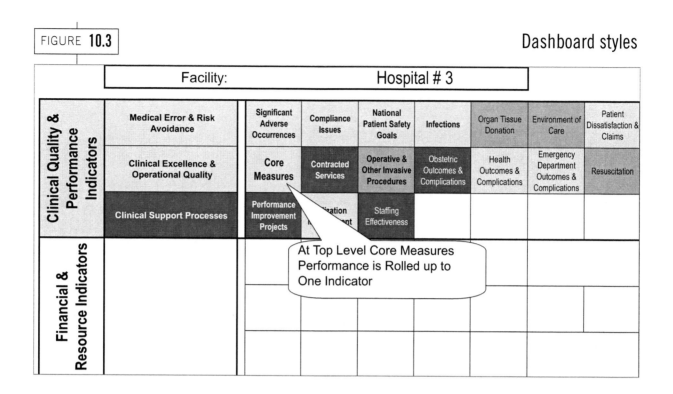

| Facility: | | Hospital # 3 | | | | | | |

Sample Level 2 dashboard

FIGURE **10.4**

| FIGURE 10.5 | | | | Sample Level 3 dashboard |

			Performance Trend			3 Month Rolling Average Comparison to Benchmark				
			12 month Rolling Average	3 Month Rolling Average	Improving or Declining?	Our System Wide	In Town Benchmark	Regional Benchmark	National Benchmark	Top 100 Hospitals
Core Measures	Acute Myocardial Infarction Prevention Process	Aspirin at Arrival	95%	88%	↓	91%	89%	91%	92%	100%
		Aspirin prescribed at discharge	100%	100%	--	100%	90%	87%	89%	100%
		ACEI or ARB for LVSD	97%	100%	↑					100%
		Adult Smoking cessation advice / counseling	94%	93%	↓					100%
		Beta Blockers prescribed at discharge	88%	80%	↓					100%
		Beta Blocker at Arrival	93%	93%	--	86%	81%	84%	86%	100%
		Fibrinolytic Therapy received within 30 minutes of Hospital Arrival	66%	80%	↑	42%	40%	26%	30%	87%
	Heart Failure	Appropriate Discharge Instructions								
		Evaluation of LVS Function					12/6/07			
		ACEI or ARB for LVSD								
		Adult Smoking cessation advice / counseling								

> At the third level all the specific details related to each of the indicators is provided.

Connecting your data to your strategy

We have now come full circle. We started with the need for data to be an important part of the control loop so that the data would change behaviors. Now, as we present our data, we want to make sure that the changes we are encouraging are consistent with the overall strategy the organization has set.

A good way to do this is to integrate all your data from the top down with the parts of the strategy that the particular indicator or piece of data supports, controls, or monitors.

Computer application vendors are making this easier with packages that help organizations integrate their measures with their strategies. Although many different vendors provide methods to integrate data, the methods we will use as an example here, provided by ActiveStrategy, Inc. offer a good model for how you might want to not only manage the presentation of your data but also to manage the performance improvement activities to cause change.

Figure 10.6 is a top-level indicator diagram of how the key types of indicators support the key strategic objectives in the hospital.

FIGURE **10.6**   Sample integration of data and indicators with strategy

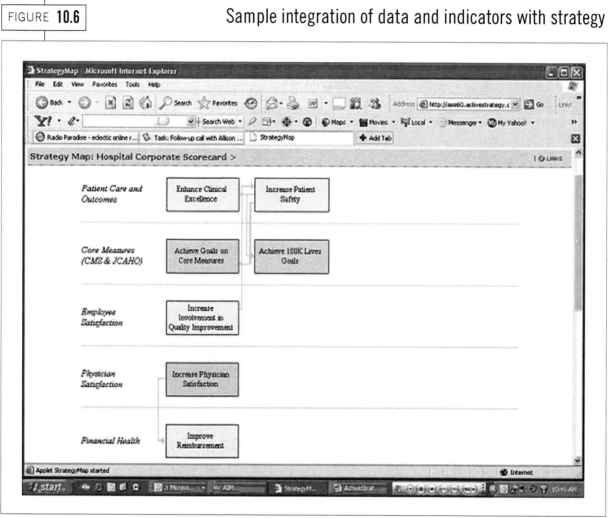

Source: ActiveStrategy, Inc. Used with permission.

Figure 10.7 shows how you can zoom in to a data book presentation that packages key information to support or diagnose the indicators. For additional detail, zoom down to the detailed data (see Figures 10.8 and 10.9). In addition, you can track the progress you are making on your improvement activities to close the loop, as shown in Figure 10.10.

FIGURE **10.7** Sample data books that package data for leadership and the board

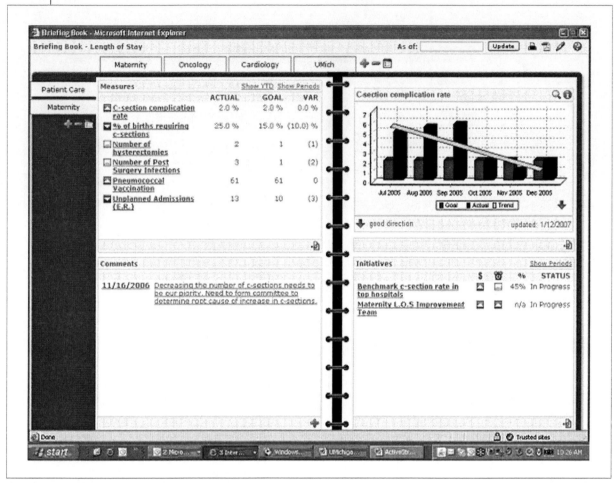

Source: ActiveStrategy, Inc. Used with permission.

FIGURE **10.8**

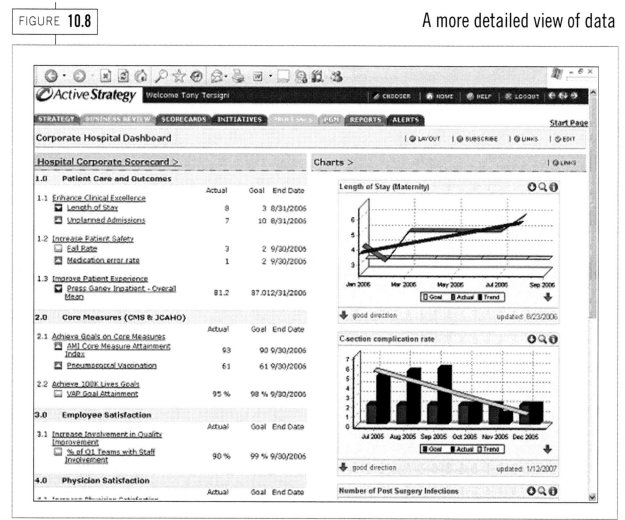

Source: ActiveStrategy, Inc. Used with permission.

FIGURE **10.9**

Detailed data graphs

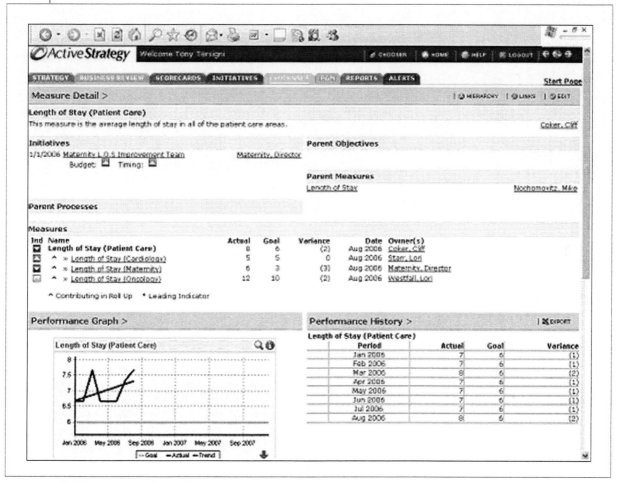

Source: ActiveStrategy, Inc. Used with permission.

FIGURE **10.10**

Closing the loop

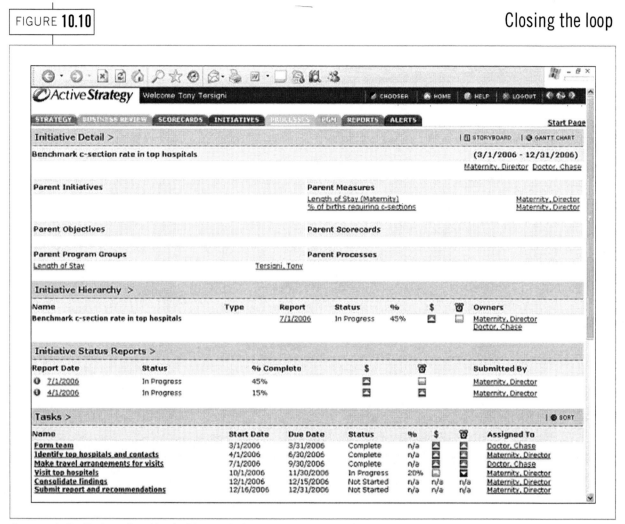

Source: ActiveStrategy, Inc. Used with permission.

CHAPTER

11

Putting it All Together

Are you ready to make your data work for you? Hopefully, the previous chapters of this book have shown you how to take some of the pain out of your data analysis and presentation efforts. Let's conclude by putting everything together. Figure 11.1 is a checklist that you can use to keep your projects moving in the right direction—from understanding *why* you're collecting data, to collection the correct data, to storing, sorting, analyzing, and presenting your findings.

The handy tip list in the Appendix is a compilation of the tips found throughout the book, and may be useful for "cutting to the chase" and staying focused. The glossary includes definitions of some of the terms and concepts we've discussed. In addition, the CD-ROM that accompanies this book includes more resources for getting the most out of your data.

FIGURE **11.1**

Chapter 11

Data checklist

Checklist for Good Data Presentation	
Do we know why we are collecting that data?	✔
Are we going to use it for immediate protection, process control or process monitoring?	✔
Is the sample frequency appropriate?	✔
Can we use the same data for other purposes?	✔
Is it "What" or "Why" data?	✔
Did we adjust it for severity or significance?	✔
Have we smoothed our data to help determine direction?	✔
Have we used crossing averages to compare our performance to ourselves?	✔
Did we use an analysis method to provide good decision support? Binning? Time series?	✔
Have we taken advantage of pivot tables and pivot charts?	✔
Did we look for underlying "Common Causes" with a Meta-analysis?	✔
Do we have regular trend meetings that are designed to produce "Ah-ha's"?	✔
Have we preplanned what we want people to do based on the data?	✔
Does the presentation method match the use to the end users?	✔
Is the data helping us or lying to us?	✔

Appendix: Resources

Tip Sheet

✔ Data that does not validate or change our behavior is not very useful.

✔ Effective data analysis and communication drives a healthy control loop.

✔ Understand the costs associated with data collection and weigh them against the cost of the problem being addressed. Do you know the cost of each data measure that is being collected?

✔ Collect data based on your processes' control needs, not based on a predetermined reporting schedule.

✔ Strive for a non-punitive data reporting process. Don't demoralize with your data.

✔ Match your data collection, analysis, and presentation to how you plan to use the data.

✔ Share your exception data between risk management and the process control functions.

✔ Healthcare facilities must use exception data (occurrence reports) to help control their processes.

✔ Remember one of the definitions of sentinel: "to observe the approach of danger, and give notice of it." Do you use your sentinel events as early warnings?

✔ You can't fix a "what"—you need to create, collect, and analyze "why" data.

✔ Always consider the severity of the event or outcomes you are counting.

✔ Always consider the normalization of your data to adjust for differences in volume, season, acuity, and so on.

✔ Look at counts, total sum of severity, and average severity when you analyze events.

✔ Develop a formal, numeric method of weighting severity.

✔ Direction, variability, and rate: Show all three in your data presentations.

✔ Monitor the goal's variability *and* its long-term rate of change.

✔ Always smooth your data to remove the variability before you try to determine direction or rate.

✔ Start simple with your analysis techniques, and build up to more sophisticated methods such as Six Sigma and advanced statistics.

✔ Know what you would do if a particular code group jumps out in a trend. The starting point is a well-designed code structure.

✔ Make sure that your coding structure allows you to roll up and roll down.

✔ If you can tell a story with your codes, they will probably help answer your questions.

✔ Goals translate drivers into action. Set your own internal goals—don't just rely on external goals.

✔ Don't limit your rallying cry goals to things you can measure.

✔ Be cautious of rallying cry goals that can backfire and demotivate.

✔ Remember, activity goals do not indicate success in changing outcomes—they just show whether you're doing what you planned.

✔ Have an emotional rallying cry goal, but demonstrate it by measurable, continuous, rate-based goals.

✔ Use crossing averages to compare short-term performance. This is useful to indicate improvement or decline.

✔ For more information, conduct a Web search on "statistical process control" or "control charts."

✔ Make sure that you know how control charts will be useful to your organization before you invest a lot of money and time in them.

✔ Don't trap yourself without a way to improve your performance!

✔ Make sure that you understand why you are putting control limits on your graphs and where they come from.

✔ You invest a lot of time and effort collecting data. Are you getting real value from your trend program?

✔ Trending causes us to "trigger" a **diagnostic** activity, which leads to a **correction** activity. Think of trending as triggering, not diagnosing.

✔ Trends look at how the direction, variability, and rate change over time.

✔ If you can't identify the number of actions the trend program has triggered, it probably isn't working well.

✔ If you can't draw a conclusion from your data, it is unlikely that others will be able to do so, either.

✔ Use your moving averages, direction indicators, and annotations to send clear messages to your leadership.

✔ Assist the departments in discovering their own "aha's" by having regularly scheduled trend review meetings.

✔ Consider your significant event data as some of the most useful and valuable information you will handle.

✔ Set up a formal process to collect the key information from each significant event and store it in the SEDB.

✔ Use some formal cutoff line to keep out of the "bug dust."

Glossary

Annotation: Explanations included in a graph to communicate (for example, the direction of the data, acceptable and unacceptable values, and a conclusion).

Binning: Sorting data sets into different categories, or bins. Putting data into bins is a natural way for us to compare data. *Binning analysis:* Comparing data via pareto charts or histograms to determine which data has the greatest contribution.

Coding: A process that identifies data and adds a value to it that can be used to bin.

Common cause analysis: investigation conducted to find underlying, common causes for trends in data; a specialized analysis of histogram or binned data to show commonalities in the results of cause analyses. Also, a meta-analysis is of many Root Cause Analyses to look for common underlying causes.

Control chart: A time series chart—sometimes called a run chart—that shows how data points deviate from the mean or center point and if they cross control limits. A control chart monitors variability in a process.

Control limits: Upper control limit (UCL): high value that, if exceeded, is cause for concern. Lower control limit (LCL): low value that, if exceeded, is cause for concern.

Control loop: The connection between the data that is collected and the system's response. In a *closed control loop*, the data feeds to the behavior and then validates it or causes the behavior to change; then that behavior feeds back into the data, which then adjusts the behavior, and so on. In a *broken control loop*, the collected data has no impact on behavior, so no change in behavior feeds back into the data.

Crossing averages: Comparison of a short-term moving average with a long-term moving average; can show a great deal about a data trend depending on which average is larger and when these averages cross.

Data: Collected, factual information that forms the basis for decision-making. *Exception data*: exceptions to a process (where ideally there would be no exceptions). Exception data tells us when something has gone wrong. *Numeric data*: parameter and specification data, usually collected in highly automated environments such as manufacturing. *Significant event data*: data related to our potentially most severe exceptions or occurrence reports (i.e., reports of medication errors, falls, treatment problems, etc.), a subset of exception data.

Moving (rolling) averages: Method in which a series of points are averaged, and that average value is used as a point on the graph.

P-chart: A chart that presents the number of defects in a data set.

Push and Pull: Two ways of delivering information. Data is "pushed" if you decide what someone needs or wants and you get the data to them. Data is "pulled" if users select and access the data they need.

Smoothing: A process that removes "spikes" in a chart or graph and therefore shows the overall direction that a project is moving.

Specification limits: Boundaries within which values or data points are acceptable. Values or data points outside of these limits are not acceptable, based on an absolute limit for acceptability.

Standard deviation: A measure of the spread of a set of data around the mean of the data.

Time series analysis: Analysis that shows how data changes over time and is used to help discover direction, variability, and rate.

Trend line: A line that fits through a set of data and shows the direction, or trend, in that data. A trend line can be a straight line or a curve, but we rely on it to determine the direction and rate of change.

Weighted significance: Values given to events or other counted data to account for differing levels of severity.